Sexual Health Information for Teens

Third Edition

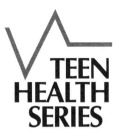

**TEEN
HEALTH
SERIES**

Third Edition

Sexual Health Information for Teens

Health Tips about Sexual Development, Reproduction, Contraception, and Sexually Transmitted Infections

Including Facts about Puberty, Sexuality, Birth Control, HIV/AIDS, Human Papillomavirus, Chlamydia, Gonorrhea, Herpes, and More

◆

Edited by Elizabeth Magill

Omnigraphics

P.O. Box 31-1640, Detroit, MI 48231

Bibliographic Note

Because this page cannot legibly accommodate all the copyright notices, the Bibliographic Note portion of the Preface constitutes an extension of the copyright notice.

Edited by Elizabeth Magill

Teen Health Series

Karen Bellenir, *Managing Editor*
David A. Cooke, MD, FACP, *Medical Consultant*
Elizabeth Collins, *Research and Permissions Coordinator*
Cherry Edwards, *Permissions Assistant*
EdIndex, Services for Publishers, *Indexers*

* * *

Omnigraphics, Inc.

Matthew P. Barbour, *Senior Vice President*
Kevin M. Hayes, *Operations Manager*

* * *

Peter E. Ruffner, *Publisher*

Copyright © 2011 Omnigraphics, Inc.
ISBN 978-0-7808-1155-3

Library of Congress Cataloging-in-Publication Data

Sexual health information for teens : health tips about sexual development, reproduction, contraception, and sexually transmitted infections : including facts about puberty, sexuality, birth control, hiv/aids, human papillomavirus, chlamydia, gonorrhea, herpes, and more / edited by Elizabeth Magill. -- 3rd ed.
   p. cm. -- (Teen health series)
   Includes bibliographical references and index.
   Summary: "Provides basic consumer health information for teens about puberty, sexuality, reproductive health, contraception, and prevention of sexually transmitted diseases. Includes index, resource information, and recommendation for further reading"--Provided by publisher.
   ISBN 978-0-7808-1155-3 (hardcover : alk. paper) 1. Teenagers--Health and hygiene. 2. Sexual health. 3. Reproductive health. 4. Puberty. 5. Sexually transmitted diseases--Prevention. 6. Sex instruction for teenagers. I. Magill, Elizabeth, 1971-
   RA777.S47 2011
   613.9'55--dc22
                                                                    2011007437

Table of Contents

Part Three: For Girls Only

Part Four: For Guys Only

Part Five: Pregnancy Prevention

Part Six: Sexually Transmitted Diseases

Part Seven: If You Need More Information

Preface

About This Book

As they mature and prepare for adulthood, teens face many academic and social challenges. In addition, they must deal with developing bodies, sexual pressures from peers, and alluring media messages. Irrespective of whether and when teens choose to enter sexual relationships, they need accurate information about how their choices can affect their health and well being.

Unplanned teen pregnancies, for example, can lead to multiple challenges. Teenagers who give birth are much more likely to deliver low birthweight or preterm infants than older women, and their babies are at elevated risk of dying in infancy. In addition, teen mothers face significant educational challenges. In fact, among women who give birth before age 18, only 66 percent graduate from high school or receive a GED, compared with 94 percent of their peers, and only two percent attain a college degree by the time they reach age 30. Furthermore, among sexually active teens and young adults, sexually transmitted infections continue to be problematic. The incidence rate for chlamydia, the most common sexually transmitted disease in the United States, has increased among 15 to 19 year olds, and human papillomavirus, which has been linked to cervical cancer risk, is also common in this age group.

Sexual Health Information for Teens, Third Edition includes reliable information that can help teens navigate the often confusing, conflicting messages they receive about sex. It also offers updated facts about the sexual issues today's teens face. It describes reproductive anatomy and the physical and emotional changes that accompany puberty and emerging sexuality, including sensitive issues such as contraception, masturbation, oral sex and sexual orientation. It offers facts about activities that can put teens at risk for unplanned pregnancies and sexually transmitted diseases. The long-term consequences of untreated, incurable sexually transmitted diseases—including cervical and other cancers, liver disease, pelvic inflammatory disease, and infertility—are also discussed. The book concludes with a directory of resources for further information and suggestions for additional reading.

How To Use This Book

This book is divided into parts and chapters. Parts focus on broad areas of interest; chapters are devoted to single topics within a part.

Part One: What To Expect As You Enter Puberty explains that confusing time in life when a person's body becomes sexually mature—a process known as puberty. It talks about male and female hormones, describes the specific changes that affect boys and girls in different ways, and provides facts about the mental changes and mood swings that often accompany puberty's physical transformations. It also discusses issues related to emerging sexuality, such as body image, gender identity, and sexual attraction.

Part Two: Protecting Your Sexual Health includes information about factors that can impact a teen's sexual health, both in the short term and the long term. It discusses sexual choices and behaviors (including the physical and emotional risks of sexual activity) and provides facts about current sexual choices among teens. In addition, it includes chapters on sexual abuse and avoiding sexual predators.

Part Three: For Girls Only begins with an anatomical review of the female reproductive system. It addresses concerns girls often have about breast development, the menstrual cycle, douching, and routine gynecological care. It also offers facts about female medical issues, including vaginal infections, toxic shock syndrome, and endometriosis.

Part Four: For Guys Only begins with an anatomical review of the male reproductive system. It addresses concerns boys often have about circumcision, penile development, nocturnal emissions, routine urological care, and testicular injuries. It also includes information about a variety of male medical issues, including testicular cancer and gynecomastia (enlarged breasts in males).

Part Five: Pregnancy Prevention offers facts about teen pregnancy and pregnancy prevention programs, including abstinence-based programs and comprehensive sex education programs. It explains different kinds of contraceptives and how to use them correctly. It also provides information on their reliability and whether or not they protect against sexually transmitted diseases.

Part Six: Sexually Transmitted Diseases includes information about chlamydia, gonorrhea, herpes, hepatitis B, syphilis, HIV/AIDS, and other diseases that are spread by sexual contact. It describes how different types of infections are transmitted, the steps that can be taken to avoid them, symptoms that may accompany infection, available treatments, and the long-term consequences associated with untreated infections and diseases for which no cure currently exists.

Part Seven: If You Need More Information offers a directory of resources and suggestions for additional information about sexual development, sexual health, and sexually transmitted diseases.

Bibliographic Note

This volume contains documents and excerpts from publications issued by the following government agencies: Centers for Disease Control and Prevention (CDC); National Cancer Institute (NCI); National Human Genome Research Institute; National Institute of Arthritis and Musculoskeletal and Skin Diseases (NIAMS); National Institute of Child Health and Human Development (NICHD); National Institute of Diabetes and Digestive and Kidney Diseases (NIDDK); U.S. Department of Health and Human Services (HHS); and U.S. Food and Drug Administration (FDA).

In addition, this volume contains copyrighted documents and articles produced by the following organizations, publications, and individuals: A.D.A.M., Inc.; Advocates for Youth; American College of Nurse-Midwives; American Social Health Association; American Urological Association Foundation; Center for Young Women's Health, Children's Hospital Boston; The Cleveland Clinic Foundation; Guttmacher Institute; Merck & Co., Inc.; National Research Center for Women and Families; Nemours Foundation;

Planned Parenthood Federation of America, Inc.; Sexuality Information and Education Council of the United States (SIECUS); and Testicular Cancer Resource Center.

The photograph on the front cover is from William Britten/iStockphoto.

Full citation information is provided on the first page of each chapter. Every effort has been made to secure all necessary rights to reprint the copyrighted material. If any omissions have been made, please contact Omnigraphics to make corrections for future editions.

Acknowledgements

In addition to the organizations listed above, special thanks are due to Liz Collins, research and permissions coordinator; Cherry Edwards, permissions assistant; Karen Bellenir, managing editor; and WhimsyInk, prepress services provider.

About the Teen Health Series

At the request of librarians serving today's young adults, the *Teen Health Series* was developed as a specially focused set of volumes within Omnigraphics' *Health Reference Series*. Each volume deals comprehensively with a topic selected according to the needs and interests of people in middle school and high school.

Teens seeking preventive guidance, information about disease warning signs, medical statistics, and risk factors for health problems will find answers to their questions in the *Teen Health Series*. The *Series*, however, is not intended to serve as a tool for diagnosing illness, in prescribing treatments, or as a substitute for the physician/patient relationship. All people concerned about medical symptoms or the possibility of disease are encouraged to seek professional care from an appropriate health care provider.

If there is a topic you would like to see addressed in a future volume of the *Teen Health Series*, please write to:

Editor
Teen Health Series
Omnigraphics, Inc.
P.O. Box 31-1640
Detroit, MI 48231

A Note about Spelling and Style

Teen Health Series editors use *Stedman's Medical Dictionary* as an authority for questions related to the spelling of medical terms and the *Chicago Manual of Style* for questions related to grammatical structures, punctuation, and other editorial concerns. Consistent adherence is not always possible, however, because the individual volumes within the *Series* include many documents from a wide variety of different producers and copyright holders, and the editor's primary goal is to present material from each source as accurately as is possible following the terms specified by each document's producer. This sometimes means that information in different chapters or sections may follow other guidelines and alternate spelling authorities. For example, occasionally a copyright holder may require that eponymous terms be shown in possessive forms (Crohn's disease *vs.* Crohn disease) or that British spelling norms be retained (leukaemia *vs.* leukemia).

Locating Information within the Teen Health Series

The *Teen Health Series* contains a wealth of information about a wide variety of medical topics. As the *Series* continues to grow in size and scope, locating the precise information needed by a specific student may become more challenging. To address this concern, information about books within the *Teen Health Series* is included in *A Contents Guide to the Health Reference Series*. The *Contents Guide* presents an extensive list of more than 15,000 diseases, treatments, and other topics of general interest compiled from the Tables of Contents and major index headings from the books of the *Teen Health Series* and *Health Reference Series*. To access *A Contents Guide to the Health Reference Series*, visit www.healthreferenceseries.com.

Our Advisory Board

We would like to thank the following advisory board members for providing guidance to the development of this *Series*:

Dr. Lynda Baker, Associate Professor of Library and Information Science, Wayne State University, Detroit, MI

Nancy Bulgarelli, William Beaumont Hospital Library, Royal Oak, MI

Karen Imarisio, Bloomfield Township Public Library,
Bloomfield Township, MI

Karen Morgan, Mardigian Library,
University of Michigan-Dearborn, Dearborn, MI

Rosemary Orlando, St. Clair Shores Public Library,
St. Clair Shores, MI

Medical Consultant

Medical consultation services are provided to the *Teen Health Series* editors by David A. Cooke, M.D. Dr. Cooke is a graduate of Brandeis University, and he received his M.D. degree from the University of Michigan. He completed residency training at the University of Wisconsin Hospital and Clinics. He is board-certified in internal medicine. Dr. Cooke currently works as part of the University of Michigan Health System and practices in Ann Arbor, MI. In his free time, he enjoys writing, science fiction, and spending time with his family.

Part One

What To Expect As You Enter Puberty

Chapter 1

Everything You Wanted To Know About Puberty

More Than A Funny Word

OK, so it's a funny word . . . but what is puberty, anyway? Puberty is the name for when your body begins to develop and change. During puberty, your body will grow faster than any other time in your life, except for when you were an infant. Back then, your body was growing rapidly and you were learning new things—you'll be doing these things and much more during puberty. Except this time, you won't have diapers or a rattle and you'll have to dress yourself!

It's good to know about the changes that come along with puberty before they happen, and it's really important to remember that everybody goes through it. No matter where you live, whether you're a guy or a girl, or whether you like hip-hop or country music, you will experience the changes that occur during puberty. No two people are exactly alike. But one thing all adults have in common is they made it through puberty.

About This Chapter: Information in this chapter is from "Everything You Wanted To Know About Puberty," May 2010, reprinted with permission from www.kidshealth.org. Copyright © 2010 The Nemours Foundation. This information was provided by Kids-Health, one of the largest resources online for medically reviewed health information written for parents, kids, and teens. For more articles like this one, visit www.KidsHealth .org, or www.TeensHealth.org.

Time To Change

When your body reaches a certain age, your brain releases a special hormone that starts the changes of puberty. It's called gonadotropin-releasing hormone, or GnRH for short. When GnRH reaches the pituitary gland (a pea-shaped gland that sits just under the brain), this gland releases into the bloodstream two more puberty hormones: luteinizing hormone (LH for short) and follicle-stimulating hormone (FSH for short). Guys and girls have both of these hormones in their bodies. And depending on whether you're a guy or a girl, these hormones go to work on different parts of the body.

For guys, these hormones travel through the blood and give the testes the signal to begin the production of testosterone and sperm. Testosterone is the hormone that causes most of the changes in a guy's body during puberty. Sperm cells must be produced for men to reproduce.

In girls, FSH and LH target the ovaries, which contain eggs that have been there since birth. The hormones stimulate the ovaries to begin producing another hormone called estrogen. Estrogen, along with FSH and LH, causes a girl's body to mature and prepares her for pregnancy.

So that's what's really happening during puberty—it's all these new chemicals moving around inside your body, turning you from a teen into an adult with adult levels of hormones.

Puberty usually starts some time between age 8 and 13 in girls and 10 and 15 in guys. Some people start puberty a bit earlier or later, though. Each person is a little different, so everyone starts and goes through puberty on his or her body's own schedule. This is one of the reasons why some of your friends might still look like kids, whereas others look more like adults.

It Doesn't Hurt . . . It's Just A Growth Spurt

"Spurt" is the word used to describe a short burst of activity, something that happens in a hurry. And a growth spurt is just that: Your body is growing, and it's happening really fast! When you enter puberty, it might seem like your sleeves are always getting shorter and your pants always look like you're ready for a flood—that's because you're experiencing a major growth spurt.

It lasts for about two to three years. When that growth spurt is at its peak, some people grow four or more inches in a year.

This growth during puberty will be the last time your body grows taller. After that, you will be at your adult height. But your height isn't the only thing that will be changing.

Taking Shape

As your body grows taller, it will change in other ways, too. You will gain weight, and as your body becomes heavier, you'll start to notice changes in its overall shape. Guys' shoulders will grow wider, and their bodies will become more muscular. Their voices will become deeper. For some guys, the breasts may grow a bit, but for most of them this growth goes away by the end of puberty.

Guys will notice other changes, too, like the lengthening and widening of the penis and the enlargement of the testes. All of these changes mean that their bodies are developing as expected during puberty.

Girls' bodies usually become curvier. They gain weight on their hips, and their breasts develop, starting with just a little swelling under the nipple. Sometimes one breast might develop more quickly than the other, but most of the time they soon even out. With all this growing and developing going on, girls will notice an increase in body fat and occasional soreness under the nipples as the breasts start to enlarge—and that's normal.

Gaining some weight is part of developing into a woman, and it's unhealthy for girls to go on a diet to try to stop this normal weight gain. If you ever have questions or concerns about your weight, talk it over with your doctor.

Usually about two to two and a half years after girls' breasts start to develop, they get their first menstrual period. This is one more thing that lets a girl know puberty is progressing and the puberty hormones have been doing their job. Girls have two ovaries, and each ovary holds thousands of eggs. During the menstrual cycle, one of the eggs comes out of an ovary and begins a trip through the fallopian tube, ending up in the uterus (the uterus is also called the womb).

Before the egg is released from the ovary, the uterus has been building up its lining with extra blood and tissue. If the egg is fertilized by a sperm cell, it stays in the uterus and grows into a baby, using that extra blood and tissue to keep it healthy and protected as it's developing.

Most of the time, though, the egg is only passing through. When the egg doesn't get fertilized, the uterus no longer needs the extra blood and tissue, so it leaves the body through the vagina as a menstrual period. A period usually lasts from five to seven days, and about two weeks after the start of the period a new egg is released, which marks the middle of each cycle.

Hair, Hair, Everywhere

Well, maybe not everywhere. But one of the first signs of puberty is hair growing where it didn't grow before. Guys and girls both begin to grow hair under their arms and in their pubic areas (on and around the genitals). It starts out looking light and sparse. Then as you go through puberty, it becomes longer, thicker, heavier, and darker. Eventually, guys also start to grow hair on their faces.

> ### ❧ It's A Fact!! Putting The P.U. In Puberty
>
> A lot of teens notice that they have a new smell under their arms and elsewhere on their bodies when they enter puberty, and it's not a pretty one. That smell is body odor, and everyone gets it. As you enter puberty, the puberty hormones affect glands in your skin, and the glands make chemicals that smell bad. These chemicals put the scent in adolescent!
>
> So what can you do to feel less stinky? Well, keeping clean is a good way to lessen the smell. You might want to take a shower every day, either in the morning before school, or the night before. Using deodorant (or deodorant with antiperspirant) every day can help keep body odor in check, too.

About Face

Another thing that comes with puberty is acne, or pimples. Acne is triggered by puberty hormones. Pimples usually start around the beginning of puberty and can stick around during adolescence (the teen years). You may notice pimples on your face, your upper back, or your upper chest. It helps to keep your skin clean, and your doctor will be able to offer some suggestions for clearing up acne. The good news about acne is that it usually gets better or disappears by the end of adolescence.

There's More?

Guys and girls will also notice other body changes as they enter puberty, and they're all normal changes. Girls might see and feel a white, mucous-like discharge from the vagina. This doesn't mean anything is wrong—it is just another sign of your changing body and hormones.

Guys will start to get erections (when the penis fills with blood and becomes hard). Erections happen when guys fantasize and think about sexual things or sometimes for no reason at all. They may experience something called nocturnal emissions (or wet dreams), when the penis becomes erect while a guy is sleeping and he ejaculates. When a guy ejaculates, semen comes out of the penis—semen is a fluid that contains sperm. That's why they're called wet dreams—they happen when you're sleeping and your underwear or the bed might be a little wet when you wake up. Wet dreams become less frequent as guys progress through puberty, and they eventually stop. Guys will also notice that their voices may "crack" and eventually get deeper.

Change Can Feel Kind Of Strange

Just as those hormones create changes in the way your body looks on the outside, they also create changes on the inside. While your body is adjusting to all the new hormones, so is your mind. During puberty, you might feel confused or have strong emotions that you've never experienced before. You may feel anxious about how your changing body looks.

You might feel overly sensitive or become easily upset. Some teens lose their tempers more than usual and get angry at their friends or families.

Sometimes it can be difficult to deal with all of these new emotions. Usually people aren't trying to hurt your feelings or upset you on purpose. It might not be your family or friends making you angry—it might be your new "puberty brain" trying to adjust. And while the adjustment can feel difficult in the beginning, it will gradually become easier. It can help to talk to someone and share the burden of how you're feeling—a friend or, even better, a parent, older sibling, or adult who's gone through it all before.

You might have new, confusing feelings about sex—and lots of questions. The adult hormones estrogen and testosterone are signals that your body is giving you new responsibilities, like the ability to create a child. That's why it's important to get all your questions answered.

It's easy to feel embarrassed or anxious when talking about sex, but you need to be sure you have all the right information. Some teens can talk to their parents about sex and get all their questions answered. But if you feel funny talking to your parents about sex, there are many other people to talk to, like your doctor, a school nurse, a teacher, a school counselor, or another adult you feel comfortable talking with.

Developing Differently

People are all a little different from one another, so it makes sense that they don't all develop in the same way. No two people are at exactly the same stage as they go through puberty, and everyone changes at his or her own pace. Some of your friends may be getting curves, whereas you don't have any yet. Maybe your best friend's voice has changed, and you think you still sound like a kid with a high, squeaky voice. Or maybe you're sick of being the tallest girl in your class or the only boy who has to shave.

But eventually everyone catches up, and the differences between you and your friends will even out. It's also good to keep in mind that there is no right or wrong way to look. That's what makes us human—we all have qualities that make us unique, on the inside and the outside.

Chapter 2

Early And Late Puberty

Precocious Puberty

Precocious puberty is puberty that begins before age eight years for girls and before age nine years for boys. The word "precocious" means developing unusually early.

Signs

The signs of precocious puberty are the same as those for regular puberty. The difference is that they start to occur at a younger age than normal.

- For females, signs include development of breasts, pubic hair, and underarm hair; increased growth rate; and menstrual bleeding.

- In boys, signs include growth of the penis and testicles, development of pubic and underarm hair, muscle growth, voice changes, and increased growth rate.

About This Chapter: Information in this chapter is from "Precocious Puberty," a document from the Eunice Kennedy Shriver National Institute of Child Health and Human Development, January 2007; and "Delayed Puberty" from the *Merck Manual of Medical Information—Home Edition*, edited by Robert S. Porter. Copyright 2008 and 2009 respectively, by Merck & Co., Inc., Whitehouse Station, NJ. Available at: http://www.merck.com/mmhe. Accessed August 2010.

Causes

Sometimes precocious puberty is the result of a structural problem in the brain that triggers puberty to begin too early. There are many conditions that may lead to precocious puberty, such as:

- congenital adrenal hyperplasia
- McCune-Albright syndrome
- gonadal (testicles or ovaries) or adrenal gland disorders or tumors
- human chorionic gonadotropin (HCG)-secreting tumors
- hypothalamic hamartoma

But in many cases, there is no identifiable cause for the precocious puberty. Puberty just starts earlier than normal. If you think your child is beginning puberty early, talk to your child's health care provider.

✎ What's It Mean?

Adrenal Glands: The part of the body responsible for releasing three different classes of hormones that control many important functions in the body. The adrenal glands are also an important source of sex steroids, such as estrogen and testosterone.

Adrenal Gland Disorders: Adrenal gland disorders occur when the adrenal glands don't work properly. Sometimes, the cause is a problem in another gland that helps to regulate the adrenal gland. In other cases, the adrenal gland itself may have the problem.

Congenital Adrenal Hyperplasia: Congenital adrenal hyperplasia, also known as CAH or 21-Hydroxylase Deficiency, is a genetic disorder of the adrenal glands.

McCune-Albright Syndrome: A disease that affects the bones, skin, and endocrine (hormone) system. It results from a change (or mutation) in a gene that occurs by chance in the womb. Because it occurs by chance, it is not inherited and passed down from one generation to the next.

Source: From "Congenital Adrenal Hyperplasia," July 2010; "McCune-Albright Syndrome," Feb. 2007; and "Adrenal Gland Disorders," July 2010, documents produced by the Eunice Kennedy Shriver National Institute of Child Health and Human Development.

Treatment

Treatment for precocious puberty can help stop puberty until the child is closer to the normal time for sexual development. One reason to consider treating precocious puberty is that rapid growth and bone maturation can prevent a child from reaching his or her full height potential.

Children grow rapidly in height during puberty and reach their final adult height after puberty. Children who go through puberty too early may not reach their full adult height potential because their growth stops too soon.

Another reason to consider treating precocious puberty is that a young child may not be psychologically ready for the physical and hormonal changes that occur in puberty.

If precocious puberty is caused by a specific medical problem, treating the underlying problem can often stop the puberty. In addition, precocious puberty can often be stopped by medical treatment to block the hormones that cause puberty.

Delayed Puberty

Delayed puberty is defined as absence of the onset of sexual maturation at the expected time.

- Some causes of delayed puberty include disorders, radiation therapy or chemotherapy, excessive dieting or exercise, genetic disorders, tumors, and certain infections.

- Typical symptoms include a lack of testicular enlargement and pubic hair in boys and a lack of breasts and a menstrual period in girls.

- The diagnosis is based on the results of a physical, various laboratory tests, a bone scan, and, if needed, a chromosomal analysis and imaging studies.

- Treatment depends on the cause and may include hormone replacement therapy or, if needed, surgery.

The onset of sexual maturation (puberty) takes place when the hypothalamus gland begins to secrete a chemical signal called gonadotropin-releasing hormone. The pituitary gland responds to this signal by releasing hormones called gonadotropins, which stimulate the growth of the sex organs (the testes in boys and the ovaries in girls). The growing sex organs secrete the sex hormones testosterone in boys and estrogen in girls. These hormones cause the development of secondary sex characteristics, including facial hair and muscle mass in boys, breasts in girls, and pubic and underarm hair and sexual desire (libido) in both sexes.

Some adolescents do not start their sexual development at the usual age. In the majority of cases, the delay represents a normal variation, which may run in the family. These adolescents have a normal growth rate and are otherwise healthy. Although the growth spurt and puberty are delayed, they eventually proceed normally.

Various disorders, such as diabetes mellitus, inflammatory bowel disease, kidney disease, cystic fibrosis, and anemia, can delay or prevent sexual development. Development may be delayed in adolescents receiving radiation therapy or cancer chemotherapy. Adolescents, particularly girls, who become very thin because of excessive exercise or dieting often have delayed puberty, including an absence of menstruation.

There are many uncommon causes of delayed puberty. Chromosomal abnormalities, such as Turner's syndrome in girls and Klinefelter's syndrome in boys, and other genetic disorders can affect production of hormones. A tumor that damages the pituitary gland or the hypothalamus can lower the levels of gonadotropins or stop production of the hormones altogether. A mumps infection can damage the testes and prevent puberty.

Symptoms

Delayed puberty is more common among boys and is defined as lack of testicular enlargement by age 14, lack of pubic hair by age 15, or a time lapse of more than five years from the start to the completion of genital enlargement. In girls, delayed puberty is defined as absence of breast development by age 13, a time lapse of more than five years from the beginning of breast growth to the first menstrual period, or failure to menstruate by age 16.

Although adolescents are typically uncomfortable about being different from their peers, boys in particular are likely to feel psychologic stress and embarrassment from delayed puberty. Girls who remain smaller and less sexually mature than their peers are not stigmatized as quickly as are boys.

Diagnosis

The initial evaluation of delayed puberty should consist of a complete history and physical, basic laboratory tests to look for signs of chronic disease, and hormone level tests. A bone age test also may be helpful. Boys under the age of 16 and girls under the age of 14 with delayed puberty who are otherwise healthy most likely have a normal or "constitutional" delay. For these adolescents, the doctor may elect to reassess at six-month intervals to ensure that puberty begins and progresses normally. Sometimes a chromosomal analysis may be performed. Girls with severely delayed puberty should be evaluated for primary amenorrhea. Computed tomography (CT) or magnetic resonance imaging (MRI) may be performed to ensure that there is no brain tumor.

Treatment

The treatment for delayed puberty depends on its cause. An adolescent who is naturally late in developing needs no treatment, although if the adolescent is severely stressed by the lack of development or development is extremely delayed, some doctors may give supplemental sex hormones to begin the process sooner. If boys show no sign of puberty or bone maturation by age 15, they may be given a four- to eight-month course of testosterone. At low doses, testosterone induces puberty, causes the development of some masculine characteristics (virilization), and does not jeopardize adult height potential. When an underlying disorder is the cause of delayed puberty, puberty usually proceeds once the disorder has been treated. Genetic disorders cannot be cured, although replacing hormones may help sex characteristics develop. Surgery may be needed for adolescents with tumors.

Chapter 3

Adolescent Medicine Specialists

What is an adolescent medicine specialist?

Zits. Periods. Pressure to do drugs, drink, or smoke. Too much growth in places you don't expect—and not so much in places you do. There's a lot going on health-wise during the teen years. It helps to have a medical team who understands.

Adolescent medicine specialists have extra training in the medical and emotional issues that many teens face. They're taught to deal with topics like reproductive health, drugs, eating disorders, irregular periods, mood changes, and problems at home or school.

Adolescent medicine specialists are doctors and other medical professionals, like nurse practitioners, who work alongside doctors to provide care.

Seeing an adolescent medicine specialist is a great way to transition from childhood—where your parents controlled your health care—to adulthood, where you need to manage your own health and well-being.

About This Chapter: Information in this chapter is from "Adolescent Medicine Specialists," June 2009, reprinted with permission from www.kidshealth.org. Copyright © 2009 The Nemours Foundation. This information was provided by KidsHealth, one of the largest resources online for medically reviewed health information written for parents, kids, and teens. For more articles like this one, visit www.KidsHealth.org, or www.TeensHealth.org.

Many adolescent medicine doctors provide gynecologic care as well, including pelvic exams when needed. So instead of seeing both a pediatrician and a gynecologist, girls often can see only an adolescent medicine doctor.

How can I find one—and what if I can't?

Start by asking your pediatrician—or your school nurse or health teacher—for recommendations on adolescent medicine specialists. Or search for one on the Society for Adolescent Medicine's online database.

It's probably easier to find an adolescent medicine specialist if you live near a large town. But don't worry if you can't find one in your area. Pediatricians, family practitioners, and internists know about teen issues too. But since they also treat non-teen patients, they may not be as focused on adolescent issues. So you might want to ask for extra time to discuss what you need when you call to book your appointment (or book the last appointment of the day). It can also help to prepare a list of questions and concerns and bring it with you to your appointment.

No matter what type of doctor you decide to see, be open and honest about the things you worry about. The only way a doctor can help you is if he or she knows what's going on. It may be hard to talk about topics like drugs you might have used or bumps "down there." But medical practitioners are used to it and they don't judge—it's all medicine to them.

A good doctor should put you at ease. If your doctor doesn't have enough time to listen to you or seems preachy, it's time to find someone who is better suited to your needs.

What's a typical visit like?

If you see an adolescent medicine doctor, you'll probably spend more time talking than you have with doctors in the past. That's especially true if it's your first visit. You might discuss things that aren't even related to why you came to see the doctor in the first place.

Talking like this helps the doctor learn about your background so he or she can tailor health advice (and treatment) to your unique needs. Depending on why you're seeing the doctor, you may have a physical exam.

Adolescent medicine specialists usually try to spend some time with their patients alone. That allows the two of you to talk about confidential issues without other family members in the room. Some doctors will let you make and go to appointments by yourself, without an adult.

Some adolescent medicine doctors have schedules that allow them to spend as much time as needed with patients. But if you have lots of questions, it can't hurt to mention that when you book your appointment.

☞ Remember!!

The teen years are one of the most crucial times for your health. It's just as important to have regular checkups now as when you were a kid to stay healthy and well, today and later in life. Adolescent medicine specialists understand that—and they're there to help!

Chapter 4

Body Image And Self-Esteem

I'm fat. I'm too skinny. I'd be happy if I were taller, shorter, had curly hair, straight hair, a smaller nose, bigger muscles, longer legs.

Do any of these statements sound familiar? Are you used to putting yourself down? If so, you're not alone. As a teen, you're going through a ton of changes in your body. And as your body changes, so does your image of yourself. Lots of people have trouble adjusting, and this can affect their self-esteem.

Why Are Self-Esteem And Body Image Important?

Self-esteem is all about how much people value themselves, the pride they feel in themselves, and how worthwhile they feel. Self-esteem is important because feeling good about yourself can affect how you act. A person who has high self-esteem will make friends easily, is more in control of his or her behavior, and will enjoy life more.

Body image is how someone feels about his or her own physical appearance.

About This Chapter: Information in this chapter is from "Body Image and Self-Esteem," May 2009, reprinted with permission from www.kidshealth.org. Copyright © 2009 The Nemours Foundation. This information was provided by KidsHealth, one of the largest resources online for medically reviewed health information written for parents, kids, and teens. For more articles like this one, visit www.KidsHealth.org, or www.TeensHealth.org.

For many people, especially those in their early teens, body image can be closely linked to self-esteem. That's because as kids develop into teens, they care more about how others see them.

What Influences A Person's Self-Esteem?

Puberty

Some teens struggle with their self-esteem when they begin puberty because the body goes through many changes. These changes, combined with a natural desire to feel accepted, mean it can be tempting for people to compare themselves with others. They may compare themselves with the people around them or with actors and celebs they see on TV, in movies, or in magazines.

But it's impossible to measure ourselves against others because the changes that come with puberty are different for everyone. Some people start developing early; others are late bloomers. Some get a temporary layer of fat to prepare for a growth spurt, others fill out permanently, and others feel like they stay skinny no matter how much they eat. It all depends on how our genes have programmed our bodies to act.

The changes that come with puberty can affect how both girls and guys feel about themselves. Some girls may feel uncomfortable or embarrassed about their maturing bodies. Others may wish that they were developing faster. Girls may feel pressure to be thin but guys may feel like they don't look big or muscular enough.

Outside Influences

It's not just development that affects self-esteem, though. Many other factors (like media images of skinny girls and bulked-up guys) can affect a person's body image too.

Family life can sometimes influence self-esteem. Some parents spend more time criticizing their kids and the way they look than praising them, which can reduce kids' ability to develop good self-esteem.

People also may experience negative comments and hurtful teasing about the way they look from classmates and peers. Sometimes racial and ethnic

prejudice is the source of such comments. Although these often come from ig-
norance, sometimes they can affect someone's body image and self-esteem.

Healthy Self-Esteem

If you have a positive body image, you probably like and accept yourself
the way you are. This healthy attitude allows you to explore other aspects of
growing up, such as developing good friendships, growing more independent
from your parents, and challenging yourself physically and mentally. Developing these parts of yourself can help boost your self-esteem.

A positive, optimistic attitude can help people develop strong self-esteem—for
example, saying, "Hey, I'm human" instead of "Wow, I'm such a loser" when you've
made a mistake, or not blaming others when things don't go as expected.

Knowing what makes you happy and how to meet your goals can help
you feel capable, strong, and in control of your life. A positive attitude and a
healthy lifestyle (such as exercising and eating right) are a great combination
for building good self-esteem.

Tips For Improving Your Body Image

Some people think they need to change how they look or act to feel good
about themselves. But actually all you need to do is change the way you see
your body and how you think about yourself.

The first thing to do is recognize that your body is your own, no matter
what shape, size, or color it comes in. If you're very worried about your weight
or size, check with your doctor to verify that things are OK. But it's no one's
business but your own what your body is like—ultimately, you have to be
happy with yourself.

Next, identify which aspects of your appearance you can realistically change
and which you can't. Everyone (even the most perfect-seeming celeb) has
things about themselves that they can't change and need to accept—like their
height, for example, or their shoe size.

If there are things about yourself that you want to change and can (such
as how fit you are), do this by making goals for yourself. For example, if you

want to get fit, make a plan to exercise every day and eat nutritious foods. Then keep track of your progress until you reach your goal. Meeting a challenge you set for yourself is a great way to boost self-esteem!

When you hear negative comments coming from within yourself, tell yourself to stop. Try building your self-esteem by giving yourself three compliments every day. While you're at it, every evening list three things in your day that really gave you pleasure. It can be anything from the way the sun felt on your face, the sound of your favorite band, or the way someone laughed at your jokes. By focusing on the good things you do and the positive aspects of your life, you can change how you feel about yourself.

Where Can I Go If I Need Help?

Sometimes low self-esteem and body image problems are too much to handle alone. A few teens may become depressed, lose interest in activities or friends—and even hurt themselves or resort to alcohol or drug abuse.

> ♣ It's A Fact!!
> **Resilience**
> People who believe in themselves are better able to recognize mistakes, learn from them, and bounce back from disappointment. This skill is called resilience.

If you're feeling this way, it can help to talk to a parent, coach, religious leader, guidance counselor, therapist, or an adult friend. A trusted adult—someone who supports you and doesn't bring you down—can help you put your body image in perspective and give you positive feedback about your body, your skills, and your abilities.

If you can't turn to anyone you know, call a teen crisis hotline (check the yellow pages under social services or search online). The most important thing is to get help if you feel like your body image and self-esteem are affecting your life.

Chapter 5

Gender And Gender Identity

Gender And Gender Identity At A Glance

- Gender is our biological, social, and legal status as girls and boys, women, and men.
- Gender identity is how you feel about and express your gender.
- Culture determines gender roles and what is masculine and feminine.

What does it mean to be a woman or man? Whether we are women or men is not determined just by our sex organs. Our gender includes a complex mix of beliefs, behaviors, and characteristics. How do you act, talk, and behave like a woman or man? Are you feminine or masculine, both, or neither? These are questions that help us get to the core of our gender and gender identity.

There are few easy answers when it comes to gender and gender identity, so it is normal to have questions. Here are some of the most common questions we hear about gender and gender identity. We hope our answers are helpful.

What Is Gender? What Is Gender Identity?

Each person has a sex, a gender, and a gender identity. These are all aspects of your sexuality. They are all about who you are, and they are all different, but related.

- Sex is biological. It includes our genetic makeup, our hormones, and our body parts, especially our sex and reproductive organs.

- Gender refers to society's expectations about how we should think and act as girls and boys, and women and men. It is our biological, social, and legal status as women and men.

- Gender identity is how we feel about and express our gender and gender roles—clothing, behavior, and personal appearance. It is a feeling that we have as early as age two or three.

What Is Feminine? What Is Masculine?

Feminine traits are ways of behaving that our culture usually associates with being a girl or woman. Masculine traits are ways of behaving that our culture usually associates with being a boy or man.

Words Commonly Used To Describe Femininity

- Dependent

- Emotional

- Passive

- Sensitive

- Quiet

- Graceful

- Innocent

- Weak

- Flirtatious

- Nurturing

- Self-critical

- Soft

- Sexually submissive

- Accepting

> ✣ **It's A Fact!!**
> **Transgender**
> Some people find that their gender identity does not match their biological sex. When this happens, the person may identify as transgender.

Words Commonly Used To Describe Masculinity

- Independent
- Non-emotional
- Aggressive
- Tough-skinned
- Competitive
- Clumsy
- Experienced
- Strong
- Active
- Self-confident
- Hard
- Sexually aggressive
- Rebellious

> ✤ **It's A Fact!!**
> **Androgyny**
> People who express masculine and feminine traits equally are sometimes called androgynous. Among androgynous people, neither masculine nor feminine traits dominate.

Clearly, society's categories for what is masculine and feminine are unrealistic. They may not capture how we truly feel, how we behave, or how we define ourselves. All men have some so-called feminine traits, and all women have some so-called masculine traits. And we may show different traits at different times. Our cultures teach women and men to be the opposite of each other in many ways. The truth is that we are more alike than different.

What Are Gender Roles?

Gender roles are the way people act, what they do and say, to express being a girl or a boy, a woman or a man. These characteristics are shaped by society. Gender roles vary greatly from one culture to the next, from one ethnic group to the next, and from one social class to another. But every culture has gender roles—they all have expectations for the way women and men, girls and boys, should dress, behave, and look.

Children learn gender roles from an early age—from their parents and family, their religion, and their culture, as well as the outside world, including television, magazines, and other media. As children grow, they adopt behaviors that are rewarded by love and praise. They stop or hide behaviors that are ridiculed, shamed, or punished. This happens early in life. By age three, children have usually learned to prefer toys and clothes that are "appropriate" to their gender.

What Are Gender Stereotypes?

A stereotype is a widely accepted judgment or bias regarding a person or group—even though it is overly simplified. Stereotypes about gender can cause unequal and unfair treatment because of a person's gender. This is called sexism.

Four Basic Kinds Of Gender Stereotypes

- *Personality Traits:* For example, women are often expected to be passive and submissive, while men are usually expected to be self-confident and aggressive.

- *Domestic Behaviors:* For example, caring for children is often considered best done by women, while household repairs are often considered best done by men.

- *Occupations:* For example, until very recently most nurses and secretaries were usually women, and most doctors and construction workers were usually men.

- *Physical Appearance:* For example, women are expected to be small and graceful, while men are expected to be tall and broad-shouldered.

Hyperfemininity And Hypermasculinity

Hyperfemininity is the exaggeration of stereotyped behavior that is believed to be feminine. Hyperfeminine women, as well as some gay men and male-to-female transgenders, exaggerate the qualities they believe to be feminine. They believe they are supposed to boost men's egos by being passive, naive, innocent, soft, flirtatious, graceful, nurturing, and accepting.

Hypermasculinity is the exaggeration of stereotyped behavior that is believed to be masculine. Hypermasculine men, as well as some lesbian and female-to-male transgenders, exaggerate the qualities they believe to be masculine. They believe they are supposed to compete with other men and dominate women by being aggressive, worldly, sexually experienced, hard, physically imposing, ambitious, and demanding.

These exaggerated gender stereotypes can create difficult relationships. Hyperfeminine women are more likely to accept physical and emotional abuse from their sex partners. Hypermasculine men are more likely to be physically and emotionally abusive to their partners.

Although most of us are not hyperfeminine or hypermasculine, many of us have anxieties and inhibitions about our femininity and masculinity.

How Can I Challenge Gender Stereotypes?

We see gender stereotypes all around us. We also may see sexism. There are ways to challenge these stereotypes to help everyone, no matter their gender or gender identity, feel equal.

- **Point It Out:** From magazines and television to film and the internet, the media is filled with negative gender stereotypes. Sometimes these stereotypes are hard to see. Talk with friends and family members about the stereotypes you see and help others recognize how sexism and gender stereotypes can hurt all of us.

- **Walk The Talk:** Be a role model for your friends and family. Respect people regardless of their gender.

- **Speak Up:** If someone is making sexist jokes, challenge them.

- **Give It A Try:** If you want to do something that is not normally associated with your gender, think about whether you'll be safe doing it. If you think you will, give it a try. People will learn from your example.

✔ Quick Tip

If you have been struggling with gender or gender identity, you're not alone. It may help you to talk to a trusted parent, friend, family member, teacher, or professional counselor.

Chapter 6

Sexual Attraction And Orientation

About Sexual Orientation

It's a natural part of life to have sexual feelings. As people pass from childhood, through adolescence, to adulthood, their sexual feelings develop and change.

During the teen years, sexual feelings are awakened in new ways because of the hormonal and physical changes of puberty. These changes involve both the body and the mind, and teens tend to wonder about new—and often intense—sexual feelings.

It takes time for many people to understand who they are and who they're becoming. Part of that understanding includes a person's sexual feelings and attractions.

The term sexual orientation refers to the gender (that is, male or female) to which a person is attracted. There are several types of sexual orientation that are commonly described:

About This Chapter: Information in this chapter is from "Sexual Attraction And Orientation," June 2009, reprinted with permission from www.kidshealth.org. Copyright © 2009 The Nemours Foundation. This information was provided by KidsHealth, one of the largest resources online for medically reviewed health information written for parents, kids, and teens. For more articles like this one, visit www.KidsHealth.org, or www.TeensHealth.org.

- **Heterosexual:** People who are heterosexual are romantically and physically attracted to members of the opposite sex: Heterosexual males are attracted to females, and heterosexual females are attracted to males. Heterosexuals are sometimes called "straight."

- **Homosexual:** People who are homosexual are romantically and physically attracted to people of the same sex: Females who are attracted to other females are lesbian; males who are attracted to other males are often known as gay. (The term gay is sometimes also used to describe homosexual individuals of either gender.)

- **Bisexual:** People who are bisexual are romantically and physically attracted to members of both sexes.

Teens—both boys and girls—often find themselves having sexual thoughts and attractions. For some, these feelings and thoughts can be intense—and even confusing or disturbing. That may be especially true for people who are having romantic or sexual thoughts about someone of the same gender. "What does that mean," they might think. "Am I gay?"

Thinking sexually about both the same sex and the opposite sex is quite common as teens sort through their emerging sexual feelings. This type of imagining about people of the same or opposite sex doesn't necessarily mean that a person fits into a particular type of sexual orientation.

Some teens may also experiment with sexual experiences, including those with members of the same sex, during the years they are exploring their own sexuality. These experiences, by themselves, do not necessarily mean that a teen is gay or straight.

Do People Choose Their Sexual Orientation?

Most medical professionals, including organizations such as the American Academy of Pediatrics (AAP) and the American Psychological Association (APA), believe that sexual orientation involves a complex mixture of biology, psychology, and environmental factors. A person's genes and inborn hormonal factors may play a role as well. These medical professionals believe that—in most cases—sexual orientation, whatever its causes, is not simply chosen.

Not everyone agrees. Some believe that individuals can choose who they are attracted to—and that people who are gay have chosen to be attracted to people of the same gender.

There are lots of opinions and stereotypes about sexual orientation. For example, having a more "feminine" appearance or interest does not mean that a teen boy is gay. And having a more "masculine" appearance doesn't mean a girl is lesbian. As with most things, making assumptions just based on looks can lead to the wrong conclusion.

It's likely that all the factors that result in someone's sexual orientation are not yet completely understood. What is certain is that people, no matter their sexual orientation, want to feel understood, respected, and accepted—particularly by their family. That's not always easy in every family.

What's It Like For Gay Teens?

For teens who are gay or lesbian, it can feel like everyone is expected to be straight. Because of this, some gay and lesbian teens may feel different from their friends when the heterosexual people around them start talking about romantic feelings, dating, and sex. They may feel like they have to pretend to feel things that they don't in order to fit. They might feel they need to deny who they are or that they have to hide an important part of themselves.

These feelings, plus fears of prejudice, can lead teens who aren't straight to keep their sexual orientation secret, even from friends and family who might be supportive. Kids and teens who are gay are likely to face people who express stereotypes, prejudices, and even hate about homosexuality.

Coming Out

Some gay or lesbian teens tell a few accepting, supportive friends and family members about their sexual orientation. This is often called coming out. Many lesbian, gay, and bisexual teens who come out to their friends and families are fully accepted by them and their communities. They feel comfortable about being attracted to someone of the same gender and don't feel particularly anxious about it.

But not everyone has the same feelings or good support systems. People who feel they need to hide who they are or who fear rejection, discrimination, or violence can be at greater risk for emotional problems like anxiety and depression.

Some gay teens without support systems can be at higher risk than heterosexual teens for dropping out of school, living on the streets, using alcohol and drugs, and even in some cases for attempting to harm themselves.

These difficulties are thought to happen more frequently not directly because they are gay, but because gay and lesbian people are more likely to be misunderstood, socially isolated, or mistreated because of their sexual orientation.

This doesn't happen to all gay teens, of course. Many gay and lesbian teens and their families have no more difficulties during the teen years than anyone else.

The Importance Of Talking

No matter what someone's sexual orientation is, learning about sexuality and relationships can be difficult for a teen to come to terms with. It can help a teen to talk to someone about the confusing feelings that go with growing up, whether it's a parent, another family member, a close friend or sibling, or a school counselor. It's not always easy for a teen to find somebody to talk to, but many of them find that confiding in someone they trust and feel close to, even if they're not completely sure how that person will react, turns out to be a positive experience.

In many communities, resources such as youth groups composed of teens who are facing similar issues can provide opportunities for people to talk to others who understand. Psychologists, psychiatrists, family doctors, and trained counselors can help teens cope—confidentially and privately—with the difficult feelings that go with their developing sexuality. These experts can also help teens to find ways to deal with any peer pressure, harassment, and bullying they may face. They can also help parents manage any complicated feelings they may be having as they come to terms with their teen's sexuality.

Whether gay, straight, bisexual, or just not sure, almost all teens have questions about reaching physical maturity and about sexual health (for example, avoiding sexually transmitted diseases). Because these can be difficult topics, it's especially important for gay and lesbian teens to find someone knowledgeable who they can trust and confide in.

Parents can help by becoming more knowledgeable about issues of sexuality—and learning to be more comfortable discussing them. Parents also can help their teen gain access to a doctor or health professional who will provide reliable health advice.

Chapter 7

Sexual Relationships

Over the course of your life, you will likely have many relationships—not all of them will be romantic, but some of them may be.

Many people begin to think about romantic relationships, or even start dating, as teenagers. People date for lots of different reasons, like to meet more friends, to have someone to hang out with, to share a new experience with someone, to be close to someone, or to be loved.

Your family and culture probably have very specific ideas about dating. In some families, teenagers are not allowed to date; others have rules about when teens can start dating, who they can see, where they can go, and what they can do. It might be helpful to talk to your parents/guardians early, so that you know what they think about dating and what their rules are.

Some teens who date may go out with someone casually, and may even date more than one person at the same time. Other teens may date one person exclusively to see if they want to enter into a more serious, romantic relationship.

About This Chapter: Information in this chapter is excerpted from "Talk About Sex," published by SIECUS, the Sexuality Information and Education Council of the United States, 90 John Street, Suite 704, New York, NY 10038, www.siecus.org. © 2005. Reprinted with permission. Reviewed by David A. Cooke, MD, FACP, October 2010. Text under the heading "Sex, the Internet, and Texting: What You Need to Know" is reprinted with permission from Planned Parenthood® Federation of America, Inc. © 2010 PPFA. All rights reserved.

The media and popular culture sometimes make it feel like we have to find our "soul mate"—the one person who can be and mean everything to us—as soon as possible. The truth is that one person can't be everything to someone else. Even people who have a romantic partner need other friends and family who care about them.

Don't give in to the pressure you may feel to find a boyfriend or girlfriend. You should know that many people prefer to hang out and share new experiences with their friends. In fact, a lot of teenagers never date. And if you do get into a relationship, don't spend all of your time with this person and ignore your friends and family.

Some dating and romantic relationships include shared sexual activity and some don't. Though it often seems like everyone is having sex—don't believe it. Many couples in dating and romantic relationships aren't having sex. Don't give in to any pressure you might feel; you have to decide what is right for you.

Communication Skills

No matter who you are talking to, good communication skills are important. How you say something can sometimes be as important as what you actually say.

Everyone has different styles of communicating. Here are some hints that might help you make sure other people understand what you are really saying.

Good Ideas

- Really listening
- Making eye contact
- Stating your feelings
- Using statements that start with "I" to show that you're talking for yourself
- Trying to understand the other person
- Offering possible solutions to a problem

- Giving positive nonverbal messages (try smiling or touching a person gently)

- Asking for clarification

Not So Good Ideas

- Not listening

- Yelling

- Blaming

- Criticizing

- Name calling

- Making the person feel guilty

- Giving negative nonverbal messages (like frowning or scowling)

- Interrupting

✤ It's A Fact!!
Communicating about sexual feelings or desires can be uncomfortable, but it is very important.

Source: © 2005 SIECUS.

Conversations about sex often involve negotiation—a way to compromise without using anger, guilt, or intimidation. People in sexual relationships may have to negotiate to set limits on sexual behaviors, decide what birth control methods they will use, and figure out how to protect themselves from sexually transmitted diseases (STDs).

To negotiate well, you have to decide what compromises you are willing to make and what choices you can't live with. It can help to identify all possible options and to imagine yourself in the other person's position.

When they are negotiating, people's styles usually fall into one of three categories: aggressive, passive, or assertive. These styles can be the difference between being mean, giving in, or being strong.

When someone is aggressive, they try to get what they want without really thinking about what the other person might want or need. This often ends up hurting someone.

When someone is passive, they go along with other people even when they don't want to.

When someone is assertive, they express what they want and feel without hurting or overpowering anyone else.

You have the right to express how you feel, to disagree with others, to ask for what you want, to refuse someone else's request, and to expect to be treated fairly without being intimidated. Being assertive can help you do this.

Sex, The Internet, And Texting: What You Need To Know

The online world gives you a seemingly limitless library of information, endless opportunities to connect with others, and all sorts of entertainment options.

And when it comes to your sex life, it can also get you into trouble.

Sexting is using cell phones to send sexy text messages or images—often of oneself. Sexting, uploading sexy pictures, and writing sexy posts online or in an e-mail may seem innocent enough, but they all actually have serious risks.

Here are some things to think about before you upload that photo to your blog or press the send button:

- **Protect your privacy.** There's no such thing as sharing information only with a select group of friends online. Anyone can forward the information to others outside the group. It's also easy to track down people through screen names, e-mail addresses, and other online profile information. And because it's so easy for people to disguise who they are on social networking sites and on e-mail, you don't always know the people you're interacting with. So never post or send anything you wouldn't want the whole world to see.

> ✔ **Quick Tip**
> Some tips on being assertive include:
> - be honest
> - be direct
> - say what you feel when you feel it rather than waiting
> - use strong body language
> - speak for yourself
> - take responsibility for your own needs and feelings
>
> Source: © 2005 SIECUS.

✤ **It's A Fact!!**

Your cell phone, IM, and social networks are all a
digital extension of who you are. When someone pressures you
or disrespects you in those places, that's not cool.

Source: © 2010 PPFA.

• **Be careful with humor.** Even if you think it's obvious that you're just
kidding, not everyone will get the joke. If you want to post or send
something that's meant to be playful—especially something sexy—make
that clear in your message.

• **Be yourself.** Your best friend thinks it would be fun to post naked
pictures of yourselves? Your boyfriend wants you to "sext" him? If you
don't feel comfortable with it, don't do it. Also be aware that, in many
places, it's illegal to send nude or semi-nude pictures of minors—even
if you are a minor, so sexting can have very serious consequences.

• **It's permanent and easily shared.** You had second thoughts about that
sexy photo you posted, so you deleted it. But someone else already copied
it and posted it to another site. And someone else downloaded it and
texted it to a friend. And somehow, it landed in your teacher's—or your
mom's—inbox. Once something is out in the online world, it's never
just a question of hitting "delete" to get rid of it.

Part Two

Protecting Your Sexual Health

Chapter 8

Facts On American Teens' Sexual And Reproductive Health

Sexual Activity

- Nearly half (46%) of all 15–19-year-olds in the United States have had sex at least once.[1]

- By age 15, only 13% of never-married teens have ever had sex. However, by the time they reach age 19, seven in 10 never-married teens have engaged in sexual intercourse.[1]

- Most young people have sex for the first time at about age 17, but they do not marry until their middle or late 20s. This means that young adults are at risk of unwanted pregnancy and sexually transmitted infections (STIs) for nearly a decade.[2]

- Teens are waiting longer to have sex than they did in the past. Some 13% of never-married females and 15% of never-married males aged 15–19 in 2002 had had sex before age 15, compared with 19% and 21%, respectively, in 1995.[1]

About This Chapter: Information in this chapter is from the Guttmacher Institute, *Facts on American teens' sexual and reproductive health, In Brief,* New York: Guttmacher Institute, 2010 http://www.guttmacher.org/pubs/FB-ATSRH.pdf, accessed August 2010.

- The majority (59%) of sexually experienced teen females had a first sexual partner who was 1–3 years their senior. Only 8% had first partners who were six or more years older.[1]

- More than three-quarters of teen females report that their first sexual experience was with a steady boyfriend, a fiancé, a husband, or a co-habiting partner.[1]

- Ten percent of young women aged 18–24 who have had sex before age 20 report that their first sex was involuntary. The younger they were at first intercourse, the higher the proportion.[1]

- Twelve percent of teen males and 10% of teen females have had heterosexual oral sex but not vaginal intercourse.[3]

- The proportion of teens who had ever had sex declined from 49% to 46% among females and from 55% to 46% among males between 1995 and 2002.[1]

% who have had intercourse, 2002

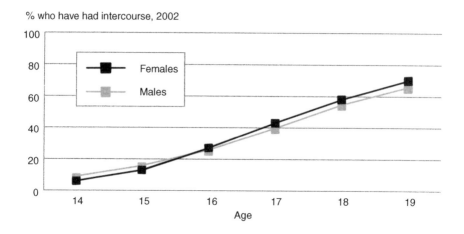

Figure 8.1. Sexual Activity. Sex is rare among very young teens, but becomes more common in the later teenage years.

Contraceptive Use

- A sexually active teen who does not use contraceptives has a 90% chance of becoming pregnant within a year.[4]

- The majority of sexually experienced teens (74% of females and 82% of males) used contraceptives the first time they had sex.[1]

- The condom is the most common contraceptive method used at first intercourse; it was used by 66% of sexually experienced females and 71% of males.[1]

- Nearly all sexually active females (98% in 2002) have used at least one method of birth control. The most common methods used are the condom (used at least once by 94%) and the pill (used at least once by 61%).[1]

- Nearly one-quarter of teens who used contraceptives the last time they had sex combined two methods, primarily the condom and a hormonal method.[1]

- At most recent sex, 83% of teen females and 91% of teen males used contraceptives. These proportions represent a marked improvement since 1995, when only 71% of teen females and 82% of teen males had used a contraceptive method at last sex.[1]

Access To Contraceptive Services

- Twenty-one states and the District of Columbia explicitly allow all minors to consent to contraceptive services without a parent's involvement (as of January 2010). Two states (Texas and Utah) require parental consent for contraceptive services in state-funded family planning programs.[5]

- Ninety percent of publicly funded family planning clinics counsel clients younger than 18 about abstinence and the importance of communicating with parents about sex.[6]

- Sixty percent of teens younger than 18 who use a clinic for sexual health services say their parents know they are there.[7]

- Among those whose parents do not know, 70% would not use the clinic to obtain prescription contraceptives if the law required that their parents be notified.[7]

- One in five teens whose parents do not know they obtain contraceptive services would continue to have sex but would either rely on withdrawal or not use any contraceptives if the law required that their parents be notified of their visit.[7]

- Only 1% of all minor adolescents who use sexual health services indicate that their only reaction to a law requiring their parents' involvement in obtaining prescription contraceptives would be to stop having sex.[7]

STIs

- Of the 18.9 million new cases of STIs each year, 9.1 million (48%) occur among 15–24-year-olds.[8]

- Although 15–24-year-olds represent only one-quarter of the sexually active population, they account for nearly half of all new STIs each year.[8]

- Human papillomavirus (HPV) infections account for about half of STIs diagnosed among 15–24-year-olds each year. HPV is extremely common, often asymptomatic, and generally harmless. However, certain types, if left undetected and untreated, can lead to cervical cancer.[8]

- In June 2006, the U.S. Food and Drug Administration approved the vaccine Gardasil as safe and effective for use among girls and women aged 9–26. The vaccine prevents infection with the types of HPV most likely to lead to cervical cancer.

Pregnancy

- Each year, almost 750,000 women aged 15–19 become pregnant. Overall, 71.5 pregnancies per 1,000 women aged 15–19 occurred in 2006; the rate declined 41% from its peak in 1990 to a low of 69.5 in 2005.[9]

- The majority of the decline in teen pregnancy rates is due to more consistent contraceptive use; the rest is due to higher proportions of teens choosing to delay sexual activity.[10]

- However, for the first time since the early 1990s, overall teen pregnancy rates increased in 2006, rising 3%. It is too soon to tell whether this reversal is simply a short-term fluctuation or the beginning of a long-term increase.[9]

- Black and Hispanic women have the highest teen pregnancy rates (126 and 127 per 1,000 women aged 15–19, respectively); non-Hispanic whites have the lowest rate (44 per 1,000).[9]

- The pregnancy rate among black teens decreased 45% between 1990 and 2005, more than the overall U.S. teen pregnancy rate declined during the same period (41%).[9]

- Eighty-two percent of teen pregnancies are unplanned; they account for about one-fifth of all unintended pregnancies annually.[11]

- Two-thirds of all teen pregnancies occur among 18–19-year-olds.[9]

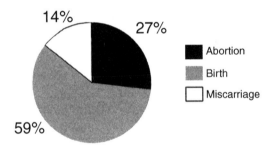

*Figure 8.2. **Teen Pregnancy Outcomes**. Nearly a third of all teen pregnancies end in abortion.*

Childbearing

- Ten percent of all U.S. births are to teens.[12]

- Fifty-nine percent of pregnancies among 15–19-year-olds ended in birth in 2006.[9]

- In 2006, there were 42 births per 1,000 women aged 15–19. The rate has dropped by 32% since 1991, when it was 62 per 1,000, but increased 4% between 2005 and 2006.[12]

- Seven percent of teen mothers receive late or no prenatal care. Babies born to teens are more likely to be low-birth-weight than are those born to women in their 20s and 30s.[12]

- Teen mothers are now more likely than in the past to complete high school or obtain a GED, but they are still less likely than women who delay childbearing to go on to college.[13]

Abortion

- There were 200,420 abortions among 15–19-year-olds in 2006.[9]

- Twenty-seven percent of pregnancies among 15–19-year-olds ended in abortion in 2006.[9]

- The reasons teens give most frequently for having an abortion are concern about how having a baby would change their lives, inability to afford a baby now, and feeling insufficiently mature to raise a child.[14]

- As of January 2010, 34 states require that a minor seeking an abortion involve her parents in the decision.[15]

- Six in 10 minors who have abortions do so with at least one parent's knowledge. The great majority of parents support their daughter's decision to have an abortion.[16]

References

1.　Abma JC et al., "Teenagers in the United States: sexual activity, contraceptive use, and childbearing, 2002," *Vital and Health Statistics*, 2004, Series 23, No. 24.

2.　The Alan Guttmacher Institute (AGI), *In Their Own Right: Addressing the Sexual and Reproductive Health Needs of American Men*, New York: AGI, 2002.

3.　Mosher WD et al., "Sexual behavior and selected health measures: men and women 15–44 years of age, United States, 2002, Advance Data" from *Vital and Health Statistics*, 2005, No. 362.

4.　Harlap S, Kost K and Forrest JD, *Preventing Pregnancy, Protecting Health: A New Look at Birth Control Choices in the United States*, New York: AGI, 1991.

5. Guttmacher Institute, "Minors' access to contraceptive services," *State Policies in Brief*, updated Jan. 1, 2010, <http://www.guttmacher.org/statecenter/spibs/spib_MACS.pdf>, accessed Jan. 26, 2010.

6. Lindberg LD et al., "Provision of contraceptive and related services by publicly funded family planning clinics, 2003," *Perspectives on Sexual and Reproductive Health*, 2006, 38(3):139–147.

7. Jones RK et al., "Adolescents' reports of parental knowledge of adolescents' use of sexual health services and their reactions to mandated parental notification for prescription contraception," *Journal of the American Medical Association*, 2005, 293(3):340–348.

8. Weinstock H et al., "Sexually transmitted diseases among American youth: incidence and prevalence estimates, 2000," *Perspectives on Sexual and Reproductive Health*, 2004, 36(1):6–10.

9. Guttmacher Institute, "U.S. Teenage Pregnancies, Births and Abortions: National and State Trends and Trends by Race and Ethnicity," accessed Jan. 26, 2010.

10. Santelli JS et al., "Explaining recent declines in adolescent pregnancy in the United States: the contribution of abstinence and improved contraceptive use," *American Journal of Public Health*, 2007, 97(1):150–156.

11. Finer LB et al., "Disparities in rates of unintended pregnancy in the United States, 1994 and 2001," *Perspectives on Sexual and Reproductive Health*, 2006, 38(2):90–96.

12. Martin JA et al., "Births: final data for 2002," *National Vital Statistics Reports*, 2003, Vol. 52, No. 10.

13. Hofferth SL et al., "The effects of early childbearing on schooling over time," *Family Planning Perspectives*, 2001, 33(6):259–267.

14. Dauphinee LA, Guttmacher Institute, New York, personal communication, Mar. 23, 2006.

15. Guttmacher Institute, "Parental involvement in minors' abortions," *State Policies in Brief*, updated Aug. 1, 2006, <http://www.guttmacher.org/statecenter/spibs/spib_PIMA.pdf>, accessed Aug. 8, 2006.

16. Henshaw SK and Kost K, "Parental involvement in minors' abortion decisions," *Family Planning Perspectives*, 1992, 24(5):196–207 & 213.

Chapter 9

Risky Sexual Behaviors

Teenagers are growing toward adulthood. Part of this transition includes learning how to handle challenging, at times difficult, situations. Teens need to have the opportunity to: explore adult roles; develop decision-making skills and independence; assume adult responsibilities; experience adult rewards; and acknowledge adult consequences.

Often this development includes risks. Risks can be good or bad, potentially healthy or unhealthy. Most teens get involved in healthy and challenging behaviors, some of which can be risky such as mountain biking, skateboarding, and extreme sports.

Preteens and teens experience significant brain growth until they reach their early to midtwenties. While this is happening, teens do not always accurately weigh the good and the bad of risks when making decisions. They need their parents and other caring adults to guide, encourage, and instruct them so they will choose healthy risks and avoid unhealthy risks.

Positive risk taking can lead to real growth and development for teens. But getting involved in unhealthy risks can lead to educational, health, and

About This Chapter: Information in this chapter is from "Risky Behaviors," and "The Emotional Risks of Early Sexual Activity," publications of the U.S. Department of Health and Human Services, August 2009; and "Sexual Risk Behaviors," a publication of the Centers for Disease Control and Prevention, August 2010.

emotional problems. Unhealthy risks include alcohol, drug, and tobacco use, sex, and violence. (Risk taking also can involve computers and the internet and video games.)

One unhealthy risk often leads to another:

- Teens who smoke are more likely to drink alcohol and use drugs.
- Teens who drink alcohol and use drugs are more likely to have sex.
- Teens who drink are seven times more likely than teens who don't to have had sex.
- Teens who use drugs are five times more likely to have had sex.

When teens were asked in a recent survey if they were drinking or using drugs the last time they had sex, almost one in four of them said yes.

♣ It's A Fact!!

In 2009, 22% of high school students who had sexual intercourse during the past three months drank alcohol or used drugs before last sexual intercourse.

Source: From "Sexual Risk Behaviors," a publication of the Centers for Disease Control and Prevention, August 2010.

The good news is that lots of teens never get involved in unhealthy and risky behaviors. The bad news is that lots do:

- Almost half (46%) of youth in grades 7–12 have never been involved in risky behaviors.
- One in four (26%) have been involved in one risky behavior.
- One in four (24%) have been involved in two to four risky behaviors.
- Four percent—or four out of every hundred teens—have been involved in five or more risky behaviors.

The other good news is that parents can help protect their teens from unhealthy behaviors. Parents who share their values and their love help protect their children.

The Emotional Risks Of Early Sexual Activity

People often believe that the only risks from teens having sex are pregnancy or getting a sexually transmitted disease (STD). Not true. Teens who have sex are at risk for emotional problems too.

It has been clear for quite some time that teen sex and emotional problems such as depression are related. What has not been clear is if teen sex causes depression, or depression causes teens to have sex. Recent research suggests that both may be true. Teens, especially girls, who have sexual intercourse may be at greater risk for depression. And depression in teens is now known to lead to risky sexual behaviors.

A 2005 study recommended that teen girls who have sex be screened for depression. This journal article found that teen girls who had sex, took drugs, and/or started drinking were up to three times more likely to be depressed a year later than girls who did not take those risks.

For boys, the researchers found things to be a bit different. Boys who do a number of unhealthy things, like smoking cigarettes every day, smoking marijuana, and drinking alcohol, were more likely to be depressed.

Another study, which also used data from that same large survey of teens, tried to learn whether depression predicts risky sexual behavior. The researchers found that boys and girls who have symptoms of depression are more likely to get involved in very risky sexual behaviors, such as not using a condom, having sex with a number of partners, and using alcohol or other drugs when they had sex.

One thing is also very clear: most teens who have sex wish they had waited. In fact, whether you ask boys or girls, older teens or younger teens, a large majority say they wish they had waited. According to a survey conducted by the National Campaign to Prevent Teen Pregnancy, two out of three (66%) sexually experienced teens wish they had waited longer before first having sexual intercourse. And nearly two out of three (63%) of those teen boys and more than two out of three (69%) of those teen girls wish they had waited. And of those teens 12–14 years old, 7 out of 10 (71%) wish they had waited. Of those teens 15–19, 6 out of 10 (63%) said they wish they had waited

Facts About Risky Behaviors

Vaginal, anal, and oral intercourse place young people at risk for human immunodeficiency virus (HIV) infection and other STDs. Vaginal intercourse carries the additional risk of pregnancy.

In the United States:

- In 2009, 46% of high school students had ever had sexual intercourse, and 14% of high school students had had four or more sex partners during their life.

- In 2009, 34% of currently sexually active high school students did not use a condom during last sexual intercourse.

- In 2002, 11% of males and females aged 15–19 had engaged in anal sex with someone of the opposite sex; 3% of males aged 15–19 had had anal sex with a male.

- In 2002, 55% of males and 54% of females aged 15–19 had engaged in oral sex with someone of the opposite sex.

- In 2006, an estimated 5,259 young people aged 13–24 in the 33 states reporting to CDC were diagnosed with HIV, representing about 14% of the persons diagnosed that year.

- Each year, there are approximately 19 million new STD infections, and almost half of them are among youth aged 15–24.

- In 2002, 12% of all pregnancies, or 757,000, occurred among adolescents aged 15–19.

> ✔ **Quick Tip**
>
> **On The Rocks**
>
> Making good sexual decisions can be complicated under the best of circumstances. If you're drunk or high, it can be nearly impossible. Alcohol and drugs get in the way of our better judgment. Staying sober is the best and safest bet.
>
> Source: Excerpted from "Talk About Sex," published by SIECUS, the Sexuality Information and Education Council of the United States, 90 John Street, Suite 704, New York, NY 10038, www.siecus.org. © 2005. Reprinted with permission. Reviewed by David A. Cooke, MD, FACP, October 2010.

Abstinence from vaginal, anal, and oral intercourse is the only 100 percent effective way to prevent HIV, other STDs, and pregnancy. The correct and consistent use of a male latex condom can reduce the risk of STD transmission, including HIV infection. However, no protective method is 100 percent effective, and condom use cannot guarantee absolute protection against any STD or pregnancy.

Chapter 10

Abuse And Rape

What are rape and date rape?

Rape is sex you don't agree to, including forcing a body part or object into your vagina, rectum (bottom), or mouth. Date rape is when you are raped by someone you know, like a boyfriend. Both are crimes. Rape is not about sex—it is an act of power by the rapist and it is always wrong.

Date rape drugs, which often have no smell or taste, can be given to you without your knowledge at parties or in a club—especially where alcohol is served. Alcohol can make you less aware of danger and make you less able to think clearly and resist sexual assault. If you are given date rape drugs, you may not be able to say "no" to unwanted sex and you may not be able to clearly remember what happened.

What is sexual assault?

Sexual assault and abuse is any kind of sexual activity that you do not agree to, including the following:

- Inappropriate touching
- Vaginal, anal, or oral sex

About This Chapter: Information in this chapter is from "What is rape and date rape?" a publication of the U.S. Department of Health and Human Services (HHS), September 2009.

- Sex that you say no to

- Rape

- Attempted rape

- Child molestation

Sexual assault can be verbal, visual, or anything that forces a person to join in unwanted sexual contact or attention. Examples of this are voyeurism (when someone watches private sexual acts), exhibitionism (when someone exposes him/herself in public), incest (sexual contact between family members), and sexual harassment. It can happen in different situations, by a stranger in an isolated place, on a date, or in the home by someone you know.

What should I know about date rape drugs?

Date rape drugs are most commonly used to sexually assault a person. The drugs often have no color, smell, or taste and are easily added to drinks without the victim's knowledge. These drugs usually cause a person to become helpless—he or she can hardly move and is not able to protect him- or herself. People who have been given date rape drugs say they felt paralyzed or couldn't see well, and had blackouts, problems talking, confusion, and dizziness. Date rape drugs can even cause death.

It's hard to know whether a party, club, or concert you plan to go to will be dangerous. Drugs may not be at every party you go to, but you should still have a plan for keeping yourself and your friends safe no matter what.

- Say NO to alcohol. Have water or soda instead.

- Open your own drinks.

- Don't let other people hand you drinks.

- Keep your drink with you at all times, even when you go to the bathroom.

- Don't share drinks.

- Don't drink from punch bowls or other large, common, open containers. They may already have drugs in them.

- Don't drink anything that tastes, looks, or smells strange. Sometimes, Gamma hydroxybutyrate (GHB) tastes salty.

- Always go to a party, club, or concert with someone you trust, such as a friend or an older brother or sister.

- Stay away from party drugs. They can be pills, liquids, or powders. These drugs can also leave you disoriented and vulnerable.

If you think that you or someone you know has been drugged and raped, remember these guidelines:

- Don't blame yourself. The rape was not your fault.

- Talk to an adult and go to the police station or hospital right away. If you don't have an adult to talk to first, just go to the police station or hospital.

- Don't urinate (pee) before getting help.

- Get a urine (pee) test as soon as possible. The drugs leave your system quickly. Rohypnol leaves your body 72 hours after you take it. GHB leaves the body in 12 hours.

✔ Quick Tip

What do I do if I am being hurt by a parent/guardian or another family member?

Sadly, there are times when different kinds of abuse happen in the home. Child abuse is when any person caring for a child fails to take care of the child, physically hurts the child, or treats the child in a sexual way. No matter what, parents, guardians, and caregivers are supposed to protect and care for their children. The term child abuse doesn't just refer to young children. Child abuse can happen to a child of any age, from infants to teenagers.

If you or someone in your family is being abused at home, call the 24-hour Childhelp National Child Abuse Hotline at 1-800-4-A-CHILD (1-800-422-4453).

Source: From "Safety in Relationships,"
U.S. Department of Health and Human Services, September 2009.

- Don't douche, bathe, or change clothes before getting help. Doing these things can remove possible evidence of the rape, such as semen (fluid from a man) or hair belonging to the person who assaulted you.

- Get medical care right away. Tell the doctor or nurse if you think you were drugged. He or she will give you a urine test right away because date rape drugs leave your body quickly. You will also get a medical exam to make sure you don't have other injuries. The doctor or nurse will test you for sexually transmitted diseases (STDs), including human immunodeficiency virus (HIV), and offer you emergency contraception to prevent pregnancy. If the doctor or nurse does not mention testing for STDs or emergency contraception, ask for them.

- The counselor will help you figure out how to tell your parents/guardians. They may be angry or upset, but only because they care about you and don't want you to get hurt. Getting help and dealing with your emotions is the first step in healing.

- You can call a crisis center or a hotline to talk with a counselor. Feelings of shame, guilt, fear, and shock are normal. It is important to get counseling from a trusted professional.

Chapter 11

Protecting Yourself From Online Sexual Predators

Is it safe to post a profile on MySpace, Friendster, or Facebook?

Many young people think the information they post on websites such as MySpace, Friendster, Facebook, blogs, or other online communities will only be seen by their friends. But, often, this is not the case. Anything you post online—even if it's in a private area—can be seen by almost anyone, including your parents/guardians, your teachers, bosses, and strangers, some of whom could be dangerous. For this reason, you should not post information about yourself. Even information that seems harmless, such as where you went to dinner last night, could be used by a stranger to find you.

You should always be careful when posting to blogs or online communities. Scam artists have been known to use personal information from your profile to pose as a friend, in hopes that you will give them more personal information, such as your credit card or cell phone numbers. Never give out ANY personal information online.

- **Before joining an online community or writing in a blog, think about who might be able to see your profile.** Some sites will let only certain users see your posted content; others let everyone see postings. Check out

About This Chapter: Information in this chapter is from "Safety in Online Communities," a publication of the U.S. Department of Health and Human Services, September 2009.

the Girls Incorporated Online Community, a safe spot to connect with your friends.

- **Think about keeping some control over the information you post.** If you can, limit access to your page to a select group of people, such as your friends from school, your club, your team, your community groups, or your family. Keep in mind, though, this does not always mean that other people can't see your page.

✔ **Quick Tip**

Be careful about posting information that could be used to identify you or locate you at home or school. This could include the name of your school, sports team, clubs, and where you work, live, or hang out.

- **Keep your information to yourself.** Don't post your full name, Social Security number, address, phone number, or bank and credit card account numbers—and don't post other people's information, either.

In some instances, you may be asked to supply your birthday or other information. For example, Facebook requests your full name, birthday, and gender in order to set up a page about you. In this case, Facebook requests your birthday to protect young people from adult content. Be sure to have an adult, like a parent or guardian, review any website that may request this kind of information before you post it. If you do receive permission from your parent or guardian to post this kind of information, be sure to limit the people who can view your information to close friends and family.

- **Make sure your screen name doesn't say too much about you.** Don't use your name, your age, or your hometown. It doesn't take a genius to combine clues to figure out who you are and where you can be found.

- **Post only information that you are comfortable with others seeing—and knowing—about you.** Many people can see your page, including your parents/guardians, your teachers, the police, the college you might want to apply to next year, or the job you might want to apply for in five years.

- **Remember that once you post information online, you can't take it back.** Even if you delete the information from a site, older versions exist on other people's computers.

☞ Remember!!

- Don't post your photo on the internet or send it to someone you don't know.

- Don't post or send personal information, including facts such as these:
  - Full name
  - Address
  - Phone number
  - Login name, IM screen name, passwords
  - School name
  - School location
  - Sports teams
  - Clubs
  - City you live in
  - Social Security number
  - Financial information (credit card numbers and bank account numbers)
  - Where you work or hang out
  - Names of family members

- **Don't post your photo.** It can be changed and spread around in ways you may not be happy about.

- **Don't flirt with strangers online.** Because some people lie about who they really are, you never really know who you're dealing with.

- **Don't meet someone you met online in person.** If someone you met online wants to meet you in person, tell your parents/guardians or a trusted adult right away.

- **Trust your gut if you have suspicions.** If you feel threatened by someone or uncomfortable because of something online, tell your parents/guardians or an adult you trust and report it to the police and the website. You could end up protecting someone else.

- **Choose your words wisely.** Some websites where you can chat with your friends have rules about what you can say. You can get kicked out if you break those rules.

Is it okay to share my password with my best friend?

No. You should not share your password with any of your friends, even your best friend. The only people who should know your internet or e-mail password are your parents/guardians and you. If you let someone else know what your password is, then they can read anything that you may want to keep private. Another person could use bad language or go to sites you shouldn't be visiting under your name.

Is there anything that I shouldn't tell someone on the internet?

Yes! Just like you wouldn't walk up to a stranger and give out your phone number or share your name, where you live, or where you go to school, you shouldn't share this kind of information online either. It is very important that you don't e-mail or IM anyone you don't know or share any information that can identify you.

Chapter 12

Sexual Choices

Talk About Sex

When it comes to sexual behavior, there are as many different possible decisions as there are people and couples. Some people feel sexual desire but don't act on it at all. Others choose to act on it alone through masturbation but decide not to be sexual with anyone else. Some people may decide to engage in some sexual behaviors but not others. The important thing is that you make the choice for yourself and stick to it.

Remember, decisions can change. You may choose to be sexual with a partner today and change your mind next week. Or you may have been sexual with a partner in the past and decide not to be with future partners. Just because you've done something before doesn't mean you have to or even should do it again—even with the same partner. Each decision is unique. So think about it.

Here are some questions to ask yourself before you engage in any sexual behavior.

About This Chapter: This chapter includes material excerpted from "Talk About Sex," published by SIECUS, the Sexuality Information and Education Council of the United States, 90 John Street, Suite 704, New York, NY 10038, www.siecus.org. © 2005. Reprinted with permission. Reviewed by David A. Cooke, MD, FACP, October 2010. The chapter also includes "Talking to Your Parents," © 2010 American Social Health Association. Reprinted with permission. For additional information, visit www.iwannaknow.org or www.ashastd.org.

Who is your partner? What is your relationship with this person? Sexual activity often involves many feelings and emotions that can be confusing. How will you and your partner handle these feelings if they come up? How will sex change your relationship with this person?

Do you feel safe? Consider your partner, the situation, the location.... Do you feel safe and taken care of? Do you feel respected by your partner? Do you respect your partner? Can you talk and listen to him/her? Are you worried that someone might walk in?

Is it consensual? No one has the right to be sexual with another person without that person's explicit permission. Have you talked about what behaviors you give permission for and have permission to start? Have you talked about where you will stop? Do you feel like your partner respects your decisions? Do you respect your partner's decisions? What is your motivation? Why are you thinking of doing this? People can have many reasons for having sex, like to become closer, to feel loved, to express love, to feel good, to satisfy curiosity, to gain popularity, to get someone to like them, to fit in, or to rebel. Let's face it, some of these aren't very good reasons for getting sexually involved with someone else. Be honest with yourself, what are your reasons?

Is it non-exploitative? Exploitation is when one person uses someone else for selfish reasons. Exploitation should not be part of sexual relationships. Partners should be interested in each other's well-being as well as their own. Are you and your partner looking out for each other?

Are you being honest? Have you talked to your partner about your feelings, what you want to do, and what you don't want to do? Were you truthful in these conversations? Being honest with yourself and your partner can help you have a better relationship.

Is it pleasurable? One reason that many people participate in various sexual activities is because these behaviors provide physical, emotional, and psychological pleasure. Does the sexual activity you are considering or engaging in feel good?

Is it protected? Most sexual behaviors carry some risk of sexually transmitted diseases (STDs) or pregnancy. It's important to protect yourself from these risks—either by avoiding behaviors and eliminating the risk or by using effective protection and reducing the risk. Do you understand the risk involved in each behavior you are considering? Do you understand the benefits of abstaining from some or all risky behaviors? Do you understand how condoms or birth control can reduce your risk? Do you know how to use condoms or birth control correctly?

What does your gut instinct say? A lot of people talk about listening to their inner voice or gut to let them know whether they are making the right decision. Think about a time that this was true for you. Maybe saying yes made you feel happy and excited or maybe it made you feel nervous and embarrassed. Maybe after you said no, you felt like a weight was lifted off your shoulders. Whatever the decision is—if it feels wrong, it is wrong for you. And remember, you can always change your mind. Even if you're in the middle of sexual activity, you can ask to stop. There is never a point of no return. You and your partner always have the right, the ability, and the responsibility to stop if either one of you changes your mind.

Unfortunately, sometimes sexual partners don't respect our wishes. See the chapter on sexual abuse for more information on date/acquaintance rape.

✔ Quick Tip

When faced with a decision try testing your gut instinct. Pick one possible choice and tell yourself it is your final decision. Keep telling yourself that for a few hours or a few days and see how you feel. Then switch to another decision. Do this as many times as there are choices. If you feel differently—whether it's better or worse—that can tell you if you're making the decision that is right for you.

Source: © 2005 SIECUS.

Sexual Behavior

Sexual feelings, fantasies, and desires are natural and you will have them throughout your life. It is possible to enjoy sexual feelings without acting on them but at various points in your life you may choose to engage in sexual behaviors.

Using the scientific or technical term to talk about a sexual behavior can feel awkward or uncomfortable and a lot of times friends and partners are going to use slang. But, learning the correct terms for different sexual behaviors can be important—it can help you understand information you find in textbooks or talk to a healthcare provider about STDs or pregnancy.

Here are a few common behaviors:

- **Abstinence:** Abstinence means choosing not to do certain things. For some people abstinence means choosing not to engage in any sexual behavior at all. Other people consider themselves abstinent as long as they haven't had vaginal sex. We define abstinence as avoiding oral, vaginal, and anal sex because these activities put you at risk for pregnancy and/or STDs.

> **✔ Quick Tip**
>
> Many sexual behaviors carry some risk for contracting STDs and some can lead to pregnancy. Check out the chapters on birth control and STDs for more information on the risks.
>
> Source: © 2005 SIECUS.

People of all ages, genders, and sexual orientations can choose to be abstinent at any time in their lives. You may choose to be abstinent for specific periods throughout your life, like when you are a teenager. Or you might decide to be abstinent until you reach certain milestones in your life like graduating from high school, finding a life-long partner, or getting married.

- **Masturbation:** Touching or rubbing your own genitals to feel good is called masturbation. Most people—male and female—have masturbated at some point in their lives. Whether you masturbate at all, and how often you do, is completely up to you. Many people are uncomfortable talking about masturbation and lots of myths still exist. You should know that masturbation causes no physical or mental harm—so don't worry about going blind or growing hair on your palms.

- **Kissing:** We pucker up all the time, whether it's giving Grandma a kiss on the cheek to say hello or brushing lips with your date to say goodnight. Obviously not all kisses are sexual, but kissing can be a sexual experience and is often the first thing that partners do together. Sexual kissing often involves open mouths and tongues and is sometimes called French kissing or making out.

- **Masturbation With A Partner:** We usually think about masturbation as something people do alone, but some people choose to touch their own genitals in front of a partner as a shared sexual experience.

- **Oral Sex:** Stimulating a partner's genitals with the mouth is called oral sex. Mouth-to-penis oral sex is sometimes referred to as fellatio and mouth-to-vulva oral sex is called cunnilingus.

- **Vaginal Intercourse:** Vaginal intercourse is putting the penis inside a partner's vagina. For many heterosexual couples this is the activity that they are talking about when they say "having sex" or "doing it." You should remember, though, that vaginal intercourse is just one of many things couples do together.

- **Anal Sex:** Putting the penis inside a partner's anus is called anal sex. Many couples (both opposite sex and same sex) choose to have anal sex.

On TV, characters tend to go from kissing good night at the door to deciding whether to have sex in just a few scenes. This can happen in real life too, but for most couples there are a lot of steps in between.

Often lumped together with terms like "fooling around" or "hooking up," these activities can be anything from giving your partner a massage, to caressing each other, touching a partner's breast, dry humping, or touching a partner's genitals. These activities may or may not lead to orgasm.

Talking To Your Parents

You probably think that talking to your parents about sex is impossible. You're not alone; 83 percent of kids your age are afraid to ask their parents about sex. Yet 51 percent of teens actually do. Why? It's a fact that teens who talk with their parents about sex are less likely to become pregnant because they're more likely to use contraception or protection when they become sexually active.

> ✔ **Quick Tip**
> ## Batter Up!
> Generations of young people have compared sex to baseball and labeled various behaviors as first, second, or third base. We all know that a baseball player has to touch second base before he can run to third. This makes it seem like there is a right way to go about sex. There isn't. Couples have to decide which behaviors they are going to engage in and then they can choose an order for themselves.
> Source: © 2005 SIECUS.

So... kids are not only talking to their parents about sex, they're also benefiting from conversations they were afraid to have in the first place! Lucky them, right? The truth is that most parents want to help their kids make smart decisions about sex. They know it's vital for teens to have accurate information and sound advice to aid the decision-making process.

Not My Parents!

Before you rule out talking to your parents, ask yourself these two questions:

- Do they want to talk about it with me, but are too nervous and embarrassed to bring it up? If you think your parents are really nervous about raising the issue, you're probably right. Many parents think that if they acknowledge their child as a sexual being, their son or daughter will think it's okay to go ahead and have sex. They might also be afraid that if they don't have all the answers, they'll look foolish. Some parents have said they're afraid kids will ask personal questions about their sex life, questions they won't want to answer.

- Do I know and trust another adult who will answer my questions without making a big deal out of it? Think about all the adults in your life. Is there someone else's parent...a teacher or guidance counselor, coach, aunt, uncle, neighbor, or another adult you instinctively trust? That's the person who will give you straight answers.

If you're still not convinced it's a good idea to talk to an adult, consider this:

- Your parents (or any other adult) are sexual beings themselves and at one time in their life, they had to make the same decisions you're struggling with right now.

- Your friends really don't know any more than you do, no matter what they say about their sexual experience.

- The internet, and other media, can't give you everything you need. Only people who know you can do that.

Now that you know why it's important to ask a caring adult about sex, you need to know how to ask the questions.

First, Set The Stage

- Try to pick a time when neither of you are in a hurry or a bad mood. "Not now" is not the answer you're shooting for.

- Choose a place that's comfortable and private. Your bedroom, the car, or a park are all good options. The idea is to minimize distractions and interruptions.

Set The Tone

- The best way to ensure that your side of the discussion will be respected, is to show respect to theirs. It's natural for you to have differing opinions; acknowledge it and respond tactfully: "I want to think more about what you've said. Can I ask you a different question?"

- Be polite. Good manners help keep the conversation on a high level of respect and can even elevate it to a higher level, especially if one of you says or does something "wrong."

- Be truthful. What's the point in asking questions if you don't want real answers? Besides, you know what happens when you're not honest. Somehow, sometime it comes back to haunt you. So just say what you mean.

- Be direct. If you want to know about birth control or sexually transmitted diseases or infections (STDs/STIs) or homosexuality or any other sensitive issue, ask. The only way to get a clear answer is to ask a question clearly.

- Listen. You might be surprised by how much they know and how good their advice is.

Choose Your Approach

- "I heard someone say..." (Fill in the blank with your question.) Then follow with: "Is that true?"

- "Some of the kids at school are doing... (Fill in the blank again.) I want to know what you think."

- "I saw this... (movie/TV show/article/ad) about... (Yup, fill in the blank again). What does it mean?"

- "What was dating like when you were my age?"

- "Did your friends try to pressure you into having sex or doing something you didn't like?"

- "Our sex-ed teacher told us about... (You know what to do here.) and I have questions I'd rather ask you."

- "I'm worried about my friend (Don't fill in the blank.) and want to help him/her. What do you think I should I do?"

- "I'm wondering what the right age is to have sex. Can we talk about it?"

Stop On A Good Note

Talking about sex with a parent or another caring adult shouldn't be a one-time, big talk. Instead, turn it into an ongoing dialog by leaving the door open for further discussion. Thank your mother, father, or whoever you talk to for taking the time to help.

And Remember: Your sexual journey is just beginning. You have time to consider your options and people to help you make healthy decisions. Take advantage of both. Be one of the "lucky" ones who listens, learns, and loves wisely.

Chapter 13

Virginity: A Very Personal Decision

Sometimes it might seem like everyone in school is talking about who's a virgin, who isn't, and who might be. For both girls and guys, the pressure can sometimes be intense.

But deciding whether it's right for you to have sex is one of the most important decisions you'll ever have to make. Each person must use his or her own judgment and decide if it's the right time—and the right person.

This means considering some very important factors—both physical ones, like the possibility of becoming pregnant or getting a sexually transmitted disease (STD)—and emotional factors, too. Though a person's body may feel ready for sex, sex also has very serious emotional consequences.

For many teens, moral factors are very important as well. Family attitudes, personal values, or religious beliefs provide them with an inner voice that guides them in resisting pressures to get sexually involved before the time is right.

About This Chapter: Information in this chapter is from "Virginity: A Very Personal Decision," April 2008, reprinted with permission from www.kidshealth.org. Copyright © 2008 The Nemours Foundation. This information was provided by KidsHealth, one of the largest resources online for medically reviewed health information written for parents, kids, and teens. For more articles like this one, visit www.KidsHealth.org, or www.TeensHealth.org.

Peer Pressure Problems And Movie Madness

Nobody wants to feel left out of things—it's natural to want to be liked and feel as if you're part of a group of friends. Unfortunately, some teens feel that they have to lose their virginity to keep up with their friends or to be accepted.

It doesn't sound like it's all that complicated; maybe most of your friends have already had sex with their boyfriends or girlfriends and act like it isn't a big deal. But sex isn't something that's only physical; it's emotional, too. And because everyone's emotions are different, it's hard to rely on your friends' opinions to decide if it's the right time for you to have sex.

What matters to you is the most important thing, and your values may not match those of your friends. That's OK—it's what makes people unique. Having sex to impress someone or to make your friends happy or feel like you have something in common with them won't make you feel very good about yourself in the long run. True friends don't really care whether a person is a virgin—they will respect your decisions, no matter what.

Even if your friends are cool with your decision, it's easy to be misled by TV shows and movies into thinking that every teen in America is having sex. Writers and producers may make a show or movie plot exciting by showing teens being sexually active, but these teens are actors, not real people with real concerns. They don't have to worry about being ready for sex, how they will feel later on, or what might happen as a result. In other words, these TV and movie plots are stories, not real life. In real life, every teen can, and should, make his or her own decision.

Boyfriend Blues Or Girlfriend Gripes

Although some teens who are going out don't pressure each other about sex, the truth is that in many relationships, one person wants to have sex although the other one doesn't.

Again, what matters most differs from person to person. Maybe one person in a relationship is more curious and has stronger sexual feelings than the other. Or another person has religious reasons why he or she doesn't want to have sex and the other person doesn't share those beliefs.

Whatever the situation, it can place stress and strain on a relationship—you want to keep your boyfriend or girlfriend happy, but you don't want to compromise what you think is right.

As with almost every other major decision in life, you need to do what is right for you and not anyone else. If you think sex is a good idea because a boyfriend or girlfriend wants to begin a sexual relationship, think again.

Anyone who tries to pressure you into having sex by saying, "if you truly cared, you wouldn't say no," or "if you loved me, you'd show it by having sex" isn't really looking out for you and what matters most to you. They're looking to satisfy their own feelings and urges about sex.

If someone says that not having sex after doing other kinds of fooling around will cause him or her physical pain, that's also a sign that that person is thinking only of himself or herself. If you feel that you should have sex because you're afraid of losing that person, it may be a good time to end the relationship.

Sex should be an expression of love—not something a person feels that he or she must do. If a boyfriend or girlfriend truly loves you, he or she won't push or pressure you to do something you don't believe in or aren't ready for yet.

Feeling Curious

You might have a lot of new sexual feelings or thoughts. These feelings and thoughts are totally normal—it means that all of your hormones are working properly. But sometimes your curiosity or sexual feelings can make you feel like it's the right time to have sex, even though it may not be.

Though your body may have the ability to have sex and you may really want to satisfy your curiosity, it doesn't mean your mind is ready. Although some teens understand how sex can affect them emotionally, many don't—and this can lead to confusion and deeply hurt feelings later.

But at the same time, don't beat yourself up or be too hard on yourself if you do have sex and then wish you hadn't. Having sexual feelings is normal and handling them can sometimes seem difficult, even if you planned otherwise. Just because you had sex once doesn't mean you have to continue or say yes later on, no matter what anyone tells you. Making mistakes is not only human, it's a major part of being a teen—and you can learn from mistakes.

Why Some Teens Wait

Some teens are waiting longer to have sex—they are thinking more carefully about what it means to lose their virginity and begin a sexual relationship.

For these teens, there are many reasons for abstinence (not having sex). Some don't want to worry about unplanned pregnancy and all its consequences. Others see abstinence as a way to protect themselves completely from STDs. Some STDs (like acquired immune deficiency syndrome, or AIDS) can literally make sex a life-or-death situation, and many teens take this very seriously.

Some teens don't have sex because their religion prohibits it or because they simply have a very strong belief system of their own. Other teens may recognize that they aren't ready emotionally and they want to wait until they're absolutely sure they can handle it.

When it comes to sex, there are two very important things to remember: one, that you are ultimately the person in charge of your own happiness and your own body; and two, you have a lot of time to wait until you're totally sure about it. If you decide to put off sex, it's OK—no matter what anyone says. Being a virgin is one of the things that proves you are in charge, and it shows that you are powerful enough to make your own decisions about your mind and body.

✔ Quick Tip

If you find yourself feeling confused about decisions related to sex, you may be able to talk to an adult (like a parent, doctor, older sibling, aunt, or uncle) for advice. Keep in mind, though, that everyone's opinion about sex is different. Even though another person may be able to share useful advice, in the end, the decision is up to you.

Part Three

For Girls Only

Chapter 14

The Female Reproductive System

Your Reproductive System: On The Inside

The ovaries are two small glands next to the uterus. The uterus (or womb) is like an inside pocket where a baby grows. Ovaries begin to make more estrogen and other hormones during puberty. This sparks the start of your menstrual cycle, which includes your period and other hormonal changes.

About once a month, the ovaries release or let go of one egg (ovum) from the one million or so eggs it has been storing since before you were born. This is called ovulation. The egg moves along a fallopian tube, which connects the ovary to the uterus. It takes around three or four days for the egg to get to the uterus. During this time, the lining of the uterus (called the endometrium) becomes thicker with blood and fluid to make itself a better home for a baby. You will get pregnant if you have sex with a male and his sperm fertilizes or joins the egg on its way to your uterus. If a fertilized egg attaches itself to the lining of the uterus, a baby may start to grow. If the egg doesn't become fertilized, it will be shed along with the lining of your uterus during your next period. The egg is too small to see.

The vagina, which is made of muscle, is a hollow canal or tube that can grow wider to deliver a baby that has finished growing inside the uterus. The opening

About This Chapter: Information in this chapter is from "How the reproductive system works," a publication of the U.S. Department of Health and Human Services, June 2008.

of the vagina is covered by the hymen, which is a thin piece of tissue that has one or more holes in it. Sometimes a hymen is stretched or torn when you use a tampon or after a first sexual experience, but this does not always happen; sometimes the hymen stays the same. If it does tear, it may bleed a little bit.

> ❖ **It's A Fact!!**
> Barrier birth control methods such as condoms can prevent sperm from passing during sexual intercourse, but these do not work 100 percent of the time.

The cervix is the narrow entryway in between the vagina and uterus. The opening of the cervix is very small, so a tampon will not slip through here and get lost. At the same time, the muscles of the cervix are flexible so that it can expand to let a baby pass through when she or he is being born.

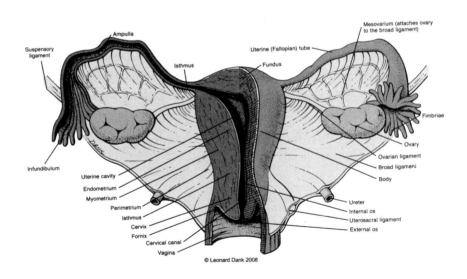

Figure 14.1. *The Female Reproductive System: On The Inside.*

Your Reproductive System: On The Outside

Outside of the body, the entrance to the vagina is covered by the vulva. The vulva has five parts: mons pubis, labia, clitoris, urinary opening, and vaginal opening.

The mons pubis is the mound of tissue and skin just below your stomach. This area becomes covered with hair when you go through puberty. The labia are the two sets of skin folds (often called lips) on either side of the opening of the vagina. The labia majora are the outer lips and the labia minora are the inner lips. The labia minora cover a small sensitive bump called the clitoris, which is at the bottom of the mons pubis. Below the clitoris is the urinary opening, which is where your urine leaves the body. Below the urinary opening is the vaginal opening, which is the entry into the vagina.

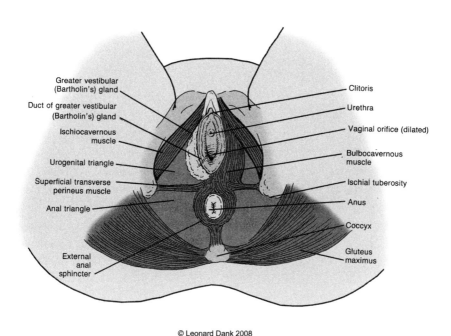

© Leonard Dank 2008

Figure 14.2. The Female Reproductive System: On The Outside.

Chapter 15

Getting Your Period (Menstruation)

Starting your period—or menstruation—is a major part of puberty and means your body now can make a baby. Usually, girls get their periods at around age 11 or 12, but it can happen any time from 8 to 16. Don't worry if you get your period later or earlier than your friends get theirs—that happens a lot. If you haven't gotten your period by 15 (or within three years of when your breasts started to grow), talk to your parent or guardian, your doctor, or another adult you trust.

Some girls find getting their periods very exciting, and others feel uncomfortable about it. It definitely can take a little getting used to! But lots of women come to see their periods as a wonderful sign that their bodies are healthy and working the way they're supposed to.

What is it?

During your period, what comes out is the blood and tissue that build up as the lining of your uterus each month. Your period flow can be light, heavy, or somewhere in between. Sometimes menstrual blood also will be different colors, like light or dark red. It may also be heavy the first day or so of your period and then decrease.

About This Chapter: Information in this chapter is from "Getting your period," a publication of the U.S. Department of Health and Human Services, October 2010.

Periods usually last between three and five days, but it is normal to have periods that are either shorter or longer. It is also normal if your periods are not the same number of days each month, especially in the first years.

How does it happen?

Your ovaries release one egg about once a month. If you have sexual intercourse, the egg can become fertilized by a man's sperm and then attach itself to the lining of the uterus and grow into a baby. If the egg does not become fertilized by sperm, the egg and the lining of your uterus (endometrium) drain out of your vagina as your period.

When does it happen?

Menstrual cycles take place over about one month (around 23 to 35 days), but each woman's cycle is different. The cycle includes not just your period, but the rise and fall of hormones and other body changes that take place over the month.

To learn about your own pattern, keep track of your periods on a calendar. Keeping track will help you to better know when to expect your next period. Also, if it usually comes on a regular schedule, you'll know if you missed one. And your gynecologist or other health care provider probably will ask when your last period was when you go for a checkup. To chart your cycle, remember that it starts with the first day of one period and goes until the first day of the next period.

How do I take care of my period?

The most commonly used products for taking care of your period are sanitary pads and tampons. You might decide one is best for you, or you may want to use a combination. No one can see that you are wearing any of the products, although you may find some pads to feel a little bulky. Try different products to find the right ones for you. Whichever ones you use, it is important to follow the instructions on the packaging and wash your hands before and after use.

You may feel nervous or shy about buying these items at the store, but getting your period is a normal part of life. Need help getting started? Ask your mom, guardian, or an older sister which sanitary products she uses. Keep in mind, you'll certainly get used to the whole experience.

✔ **Quick Tip**

Keep in mind that at first, your periods may not be regular;
you may have two in one month, or have a month without a period at all.
Periods will become more regular in time.

What should I know about pads?

- Pads stick to the inside of your underwear and soak up the blood that leaves the vagina.

- Some pads are thinner for days when your period is light, and some are thicker for when you are bleeding more. You can also use these thicker pads at night when you sleep.

- During the day, it is best to check your pad to see if it needs changing every couple of hours. You should change it before it is soaked with blood.

- If you are concerned about any smell, changing pads often and keeping up good hygiene will help control this. You do not need to use deodorant pads (and sometimes they can be irritating).

- You can use a panty liner, which is a very thin pad, together with a tampon if you want extra protection. Or you can use a liner alone on light days.

- You probably don't want to wear pads when you swim. They will soak up water and be bulky. You could try a tampon instead.

What should I know about tampons?

- Tampons are put inside your vagina to soak up blood before it leaves your body. Instructions come with tampon products to show you how to put them in. It sometimes takes practice.

- Some tampons have a plastic or cardboard covering that makes it easier for you to put the tampon in. This is called the applicator. Do not leave the applicator inside your vagina.

- All tampons have a string at the end to help you take it out when it needs to be changed (at least every four to eight hours).

- Tampons will not get lost in your vagina or "slip up."

- You can wear tampons when you swim. Water does not enter your vagina.

- If you have trouble putting in a tampon, you might try a smaller one or one with an applicator. If you really cannot get it in, you might see your doctor.

- It is very important that you use the tampon with the lowest level of absorbency for your needs. On the heavy days, you may need a super tampon and as your flow gets lighter, you may only need a regular tampon. Or, you may only need a regular tampon on your heavy days, and then can switch to a junior tampon for your lighter days. You will be able to tell what level of absorbency you need by how often you need to change your tampon.

- Using tampons that are too absorbent or not changing them often enough can put you at risk of TSS. You can avoid TSS by not using tampons at all, changing them often, or by switching back and forth between tampons and pads. While the symptoms of TSS can be caused by many other illnesses, tell an adult and call a doctor if you are using tampons and have the following:

  - High fever that comes on all of a sudden

  - Muscle pains

  - Dizziness or fainting

  - A rash that looks like sunburn

  - Redness of eyes, mouth, and throat

  - Strange vaginal discharge (fluid)

  - A feeling of confusion

> ♣ **It's A Fact!!**
> **What is**
> **toxic shock**
> **syndrome (TSS)?**
>
> TSS is a very rare but dangerous illness that affects your whole body. TSS is caused by certain types of bacteria that make poisons in your body. Tampons may make it easier for bacteria to grow in your body. It is also possible to get TSS if bacteria get into an open wound. Make sure you clean all skin wounds and infections well, with the help of a parent or guardian.

✔ **Quick Tip**

Doctors treat TSS with antibiotics, and will examine
your kidneys and liver to make sure they are working okay.
Doctors will also treat your rash to help you heal. It is important to
get medical help right away if you have any of the symptoms
described in this chapter.

How else can I care for my period?

Chances are good that you've seen tampons and sanitary pads, but you
may not know about alternative care products that are natural or reusable.
Some girls choose items like menstrual cups or reusable pads because they
feel they are better for their bodies and for the environment. If you're interested in trying some, you may find them in your local supermarket or
drugstore. If not, you can go to a natural foods store or buy them online.
Here are some options:

- **Menstrual Cups:** This is a small cup that is put inside the vagina to
  collect blood. Some cups are for one-time use. Others are emptied,
  washed well, and reused.

- **Reusable Pads:** These are pads that are washed and reused. Usually,
  you would put a cloth pad into a liner that attaches to your underwear.
  You change the pad as needed and wash it according to the maker's
  instructions. These pads are more expensive to buy than disposable ones,
  but they save money over time because they last for years.

- **Reusable Menstrual Sponges:** These are natural sponges from the
  ocean floor. They work the same way tampons do. You need to change
  them around every four to six hours and wash them well. Just like with
  regular tampons, it may be possible to get TSS from sea sponges.

- **Non-Chlorine Bleached All-Cotton Pads And Tampons:** These are
  disposable like regular tampons and pads, but they aren't made using
  chemicals.

Chapter 16

Problems With Your Period

Being uncomfortable or having cramps along with your period is very common. It is also common for your periods to be irregular sometimes, meaning you may not get it at the same time each month or at all some months. These things can happen and there may not necessarily be a problem, even though you might be uncomfortable or in pain. The tough thing is knowing when the things you are feeling are normal and when there is a problem. To make this easier, get to know yourself:

- How painful are your cramps each month? If you start to have cramps that are much worse than usual, talk to your parents/guardian about seeing a doctor.

- What days of the month do you get your period? How long does it last?

- What is your stress level like when you get your period? Are you a little more stressed around the time of your period, or do you feel like you can't cope at all with school and family issues?

- How heavy is your blood flow? You can tell how heavy it is by how many times you have to change your pads or tampons.

About This Chapter: Information in this chapter is from "Problem periods," a publication of the U.S. Department of Health and Human Services, June 2008.

Answering these questions can help you figure out what your periods are usually like. If you are in pain or are not sure if what is happening with your period is a problem or not, talk with your parents/guardian about making an appointment to see your doctor. And having answers to the questions above can help you talk to your doctor about what you are dealing with.

Factors That Can Affect Your Period
Stress

If you are under a lot of stress, your periods might stop for a bit, but they usually begin again when your stress level goes down.

Exercise

Too much exercise can cause your body fat to be very low, which can cause your periods to stop. This can happen if you are training hard for sports such as ballet, gymnastics, or long-distance running. It can also happen if you are exercising a lot in other ways on your own. It might seem confusing, since you often hear that exercise is good for you. It is good for you—as long as you don't overexercise. How do you know if you are exercising too much? If you are overtired or get injured often, you may be overdoing it.

Hormones

Hormones are special chemicals that your body makes. In a normal menstrual cycle, your hormones go up and down. Sometimes there are problems with hormones. A hormonal imbalance called polycystic ovary syndrome (PCOS) keeps your hormone levels high, getting in the way of your cycle. If you have PCOS, your periods may not come every month, they may not come at all, or you may have bleeding in between periods.

✔ **Quick Tip**
Even though PMS and dysmenorrhea can be a normal part of having your period, be sure to see your doctor for tips on feeling better and to make sure you do not have a serious health problem.

A problem with your pituitary gland can also affect your menstrual cycle. The pituitary gland makes hormones that impact other glands in the endocrine system (the body system that controls growth, sexual development, and metabolism).

When To See A Doctor

You should talk to an adult you trust and/or see a doctor if you experience any of the following:

- You have not gotten your period by the age of 16

- Your period suddenly stops, and it has been three to six months and it hasn't started again (and you know you aren't pregnant, confirmed by a doctor's pregnancy test or by not having had sexual intercourse)

- You are bleeding for more days than usual (abnormal bleeding that is different from your normal menstrual periods)

- Your bleeding is very heavy (abnormal bleeding that is different from your normal menstrual periods)

- You suddenly feel sick after using tampons

- You bleed in between periods (more than just a few drops)

Common Period Problems

You're 16, But Haven't Gotten Your Period Yet

If you have not started your period and it has been five or more years since your breasts first started to grow, you could be dealing with delayed (late) puberty. If you are 16 or older, talk to your parents/guardian about seeing a doctor. Sometimes there is a medical reason for delayed puberty, such as poor nutrition, but there is no cause for most women and no treatment is needed. Puberty will happen in time.

Not having regular periods (one each month) can be a sign of PCOS, which can cause you to miss periods, stop getting your period, or have bleeding at times when you aren't supposed to have your period. PCOS can also cause weight gain, a lot of facial hair, pain in your pelvic area, bad acne, and dandruff (white flakes in your hair). Only a doctor can tell you if you have PCOS.

Your Period Doesn't Follow A Schedule At All

When you first get your period, it is normal to have some months when you don't have a period, or even months when you have two periods. They should become more regular (once a month) over time. If this does not happen, you may have PCOS.

Your Cramps Are Horrible

You may have premenstrual syndrome (PMS) or dysmenorrhea, painful cramps caused by abnormal muscle movements in your uterus during periods. Things that can put you at risk for dysmenorrhea include smoking, being overweight, and starting your period before age 11. Other signs of dysmenorrhea are: pain down your legs, throwing up, diarrhea, being tired, weakness, fainting, and headaches. Only a doctor can tell you if you have dysmenorrhea.

Painful cramps can be a sign of endometriosis, a common disease among women. (About 5.5 million women in the U.S. have it.) Endometriosis happens when tissue that is supposed to grow in the uterus makes its way to grow in other parts of your pelvic and lower stomach areas. Along with cramps, endometriosis can also cause heavy periods, long lasting pain in your pelvic area, and lower back pain. For many women, endometriosis can be treated with medicines or surgery. Only a doctor can tell you if you have endometriosis.

Painful cramps can also be a sign of an infection such as pelvic inflammatory disease or PID. PID is commonly caused by chlamydia and gonorrhea, diseases passed on through sexual contact. If you have pain in your lower stomach, bleeding in between periods, or fluid coming from your vagina that has a bad odor, see your doctor right away for treatment. If you do not treat PID, it can damage your fallopian tubes and hurt your ability

> **✔ Quick Tip**
>
> While amenorrhea may be caused by a health problem that needs to be treated, there are some things you can do to try to keep your periods on a regular schedule: keep a healthy body weight for your height; ask your parents/guardian or doctor for help controlling stress if you feel overwhelmed; stay away from drugs and alcohol; and don't smoke.

to have babies later in life. The only way to totally avoid PID caused by sexually transmitted infections is to avoid sex. Condoms can help prevent sexually transmitted infections, but it is still possible for the germs to pass from one person to another when there is sexual contact.

You Are No Longer Getting Your Period

When you stop getting your period, it is called amenorrhea. If you have had sexual intercourse, you will first need to see your doctor to find out if you are pregnant. If you know you are not pregnant and have not had your period for three to six months, you will need to see your doctor to find out why your periods have stopped and to fix the problem. The following things can cause your period to stop: eating disorders; overexercising; stress; certain medicines (chemotherapy, used to treat cancer, and some antidepressants, used to treat depression and other health problems); problems with your thyroid; and PCOS.

Your Period Is Really Heavy

Heavy periods can be a sign of endometriosis, a common disease among women.

You might also want to talk with your doctor about a bleeding disorder (problem) if you have very heavy menstrual periods, especially starting with your first period. You should also talk to the doctor if you have had problems with the following: easy bruising; nosebleeds that last a long time and happen often; or heavy bleeding that lasts a long time after minor cuts, dental work, or surgery.

The most common bleeding problem in girls and women is von Willebrand's disease or VWD. People who have this disease are missing something in the blood that helps you clot normally, or stop bleeding. This disorder runs in families, so your mother, sister, female cousins, or aunts also might have some of the signs listed above. To find out if you have this disorder, you will need special blood tests to check for von Willebrand's and to find out your blood type. Your test results can be wrong if you're taking hormones—which can be used to treat heavy bleeding—so it is best to have the test done before getting treated.

You Have Acne Or A Lot Of Facial Hair

Having acne is a normal part of being a teen. If you have bad acne on top of irregular periods, a lot of facial hair, weight gain, and pelvic pain, you may have PCOS.

Chapter 17

Breast Health

Mammograms And Breast Health

Women's breasts come in all shapes and sizes. There is no perfect shape or size for breasts. Normal breasts can be large or small, smooth or lumpy, and light or dark. Most young women have a lot of questions about their breasts.

How do breasts develop?

The inside of your breasts is made up of fatty tissue and many milk-producing glands, called mammary glands. The dark area of your breast around your nipple is called the areola. As your body starts to develop, a small bump grows under the areola and nipple. This bump is called the breast bud. As the buds get larger and rounder, the breasts grow. As your breasts develop, the areolae get bigger and darker. Areolae and nipples can range in color from light pink to purplish to light gray depending on your skin color.

About This Chapter: This chapter begins with information from "Mammograms & Breast Health: An Information Guide for Women," a publication of the Centers for Disease Control and Prevention, March 2006. The end of the chapter presents material excerpted from "Teens And Breast Implants," © 2010 National Research Center for Women and Families. Reprinted with permission. The complete text of this document including references is available at http://www.breastimplantinfo.org/news/teen_implants.html. For additional information, visit www.breastimplantinfo.org or www.center4research.org.

When will I get breasts?

Your breasts start growing when you begin puberty. Puberty is the name for the time when your body goes through changes and you begin to go from being a child to an adult. During puberty the hormone levels in your body change, causing your breasts to develop and your menstrual periods to start. Heredity (the way certain characteristics are passed down from generation to generation) and nutrition determine when you are going to begin puberty and develop breasts. Most girls' breasts begin growing when they are about 10 or 11 years old, but some girls may start developing breasts earlier or later than this age.

How long will it take to get breasts?

It takes three to five years from the time your breasts start growing until they reach their full size. The age when you start to develop does not have an effect on the final size of your breasts. For example, if you develop earlier than most girls, this doesn't mean that you will have bigger breasts than most girls.

Is there anything I can do to increase the size of my breasts?

Heredity is the most important factor in determining breast shape and size. No creams, special exercises, or clothing will permanently change your breast size. Your breasts may change with weight loss or gain or after a pregnancy, but for the most part the size of your breasts stays the same once you have finished puberty. Also, breast size has no effect on whether a woman will be able to breastfeed her baby.

When and how will my breasts make milk?

Inside a woman's breasts are tiny pockets called alveoli. After a woman gives birth, her brain's hormones tell the alveoli to produce milk. When her baby sucks on her nipple, the sucking draws milk from the alveoli through the milk ducts and out small holes in the nipple. When the mother stops breastfeeding her baby, her alveoli slowly stop making milk.

My breasts are uneven. Is this normal?

It is very common for your breasts to grow at different rates while they're developing. Usually, they will look about the same size by the time they are done growing. If the size difference bothers you, you can try foam or gel inserts that fit into your bra or bathing suit. These inserts are sold at specialty bra and lingerie shops.

My breasts are very large, and they make my back hurt because they're so heavy. It's also hard to exercise, because I get sore breasts. What can I do?

If your breasts are very large, there are some options that can help:

- First, find a well-fitting bra to minimize and support your breasts. Look for a bra that has wide shoulder straps and supportive cups. If you need help with measuring for a bra, see a trained salesperson working at a department store or a lingerie store for help.

- If you are overweight, working to reach a healthy weight may also help.

- The last option is to have a breast reduction surgery. This type of surgery, which is done by a plastic surgeon, removes some of the extra breast tissue to decrease pain. It is a big surgery, and you should talk about it with your health care provider.

Is breast pain or tenderness normal?

You may feel a tingling or aching in your chest when your breast buds start developing. After you start to get your periods you may notice that your breasts become tender or sore about a week before you get your period each month. This soreness does not happen to everyone. If you are having pain, check with your health care provider who may suggest taking medication (such as ibuprofen) to help with the symptoms.

Is it normal to have lumpy breasts?

Normal breasts can be smooth or lumpy. Most lumps are due to normal changes in breast tissue that occur during development. Your breasts may also feel different or lumpy around the time of your period. If you do notice that a new lump appears in your breast and does not disappear after your period, you should contact your health care provider.

✤ It's A Fact!!

Buying A Bra

If you are about to buy your first bra, it's best to go to a department store that has a special department that sells bras and underwear, usually called the lingerie department. Ask to be fitted by a lingerie specialist (a professional who has special training in fitting bras). This service is free, and having the measurements done by a professional will make sure that your bra fits correctly.

If you prefer to measure yourself at home, place a cloth measuring tape under your breasts. Wrap the tape around your chest so the tape measure meets the beginning part of the tape. When you have the measurement number, add five inches. For example, if your measurement around your chest is 27 inches, your chest size is 32.

If your measurement is an ODD number, you will need to go up to the next EVEN number to figure out your size. For example, if your chest measurement is 28 inches, your chest size is 34.

Source: From Centers for Disease Control and Prevention, March 2006.

Who is at risk for breast cancer?

Women with certain medical conditions, lifestyle habits, or traits (referred to as risk factors) may be more likely than other women to get cancer. However, having risk factors does not mean you will get breast cancer. Most women who develop breast cancer have no risk factors at all. Overall, you are at a higher risk for developing breast cancer if you have these characteristics:

- Have close relatives (mother, sister, grandmother, or aunt) who have had breast cancer

- Are obese

- Drink alcohol excessively

How can I lower my risk for breast cancer?

You can lower your risk for breast cancer by keeping your lifestyle healthy. Don't smoke, limit alcohol intake, exercise regularly, follow a healthy diet, and have regular checkups with your health care provider.

Do I need to have a mammogram?

A mammogram is an x-ray of the breasts, usually done to try to find early signs of breast cancer. Teens do not need to get mammograms.

Teens And Breast Implants

- According to the American Society of Plastic Surgeons, more than 209,000 teenagers underwent plastic surgery and cosmetic procedures in 2009. Most were nonsurgical procedures such as laser hair removal and laser skin resurfacing, but breast augmentation was one of the most popular surgeries.

- Breast augmentation has become a frequently-requested high school graduation gift. How frequently is it requested or given as a gift? Nobody really knows, since the research has not been done.

- Is it appropriate to perform cosmetic surgery on patients whose bodies are still maturing? Breast development can continue into the late teens and early twenties, so girls who think they need augmentation now might change their mind later.

- There are no epidemiological studies or clinical trials on the safety and long-term risks of breast implants and liposuction on patients under 18. So, the risks are unknown.

- Although the Food and Drug Administration (FDA) approved silicone gel breast implants only for women ages 21 and older, and saline breast implants only for women 18 and older, there are no legal restrictions on the procedure. The American Society of Plastic Surgeons has an official position against breast augmentation for most teens under 18, but there is no enforcement. The American Society for Aesthetic Plastic Surgeons has no official position regarding augmentation for teenagers

✣ **It's A Fact!!**
Your health care provider will perform a breast exam once a year. While you may find this a little embarrassing, a breast exam is an important way for your health care provider to learn what is normal for your breasts and to find any lumps that aren't normal.

Source: From Centers for Disease Control and Prevention, March 2006.

- Research has shown that of all age groups, teenagers are the most likely to be dissatisfied with their appearance—and that the dissatisfaction lessens with age. A long-term study conducted on both boys and girls ages 11–18 found that body image satisfaction was highest at age 18 for both boys and girls. In other words, older teens feel better about their bodies than younger teens. The study also found that the features participants were most dissatisfied with reflected the culturally determined stereotypes emphasized in books, mass media, and advertisements.

- Breast augmentation has a very high complication rate that often requires additional surgery within five to 10 years. For a girl of 18, that means she will probably need another surgery while she is in her 20s, her 30s, and every decade after that.

- Based on the implant makers' own studies, the FDA concluded that about 40 percent of augmentation patients have at least one serious complication within three years after getting their saline implants.

- Breast pain, breast hardness, and numbness in the nipple area are common complications that may last for years, and may never go away.

- According to studies by the National Cancer Institute and other researchers, breast augmentation patients are four times more likely to commit suicide compared to other women of the same age, including former plastic surgery patients of the same age. The risk of lung cancer and some other cancers also is higher for breast augmentation patients compared to similar women without implants.

- Health insurance usually will not pay for the necessary treatment or corrective surgeries for breast implant problems. Teens may not think about their future financial security, since their main concern is the immediate gratification of fixing a perceived problem with their bodies. But fixing implant problems costs thousands of dollars each time, so these financial considerations are important.

- Breast implants interfere with mammography, hiding 55 percent of breast tumors, on average.

- Breast implant surgery sometimes causes infections leading to toxic shock syndrome, amputation, or death.

- Women who have breast implants are less likely to have enough milk to be able to breastfeed, compared to women who have not had breast surgery.

- If a teenager changes her mind and has her implants removed a few years later, her breasts are likely to look stretched out and saggy. This is especially true for women with larger implants.

Chapter 18

When To See A Gynecologist

When do I need to go?

A gynecologist is a doctor who has been specially trained in women's reproductive health issues. You should talk to a parent or guardian about seeing a gynecologist (or another doctor who is specially trained in women's health issues) if these characteristics apply to you:

- Have ever had sex (vaginal, oral or anal) or intimate sexual contact

- Are 21 or older

- Have lower stomach pain, fever, and discharge (fluid coming from your vagina) that is yellow, gray, or green with a strong smell. These may be symptoms of pelvic inflammatory disease (PID). PID is a general term for an infection of the lining of the uterus, fallopian tubes, or the ovaries. Most of the time, PID is caused by sexually transmitted infections (STIs) such as chlamydia and gonorrhea that have not been treated. Not all vaginal discharges are symptoms of sexually transmitted infections.

After your first checkup, your doctor will tell you when it is time to come back for another visit.

About This Chapter: Information in this chapter is from "When to see a gynecologist," a publication of the U.S. Department of Health and Human Services, June 2008.

Why do I need to go?

Getting routine gynecology care will establish what is normal for you. It will also help you: understand your body and how it works; find problems early so they can be treated or kept from getting worse; understand why it's healthier for you not to have sex while you are a teenager; learn how to protect yourself if you do have sex; and prepare for healthy relationships and future pregnancies.

> ♣ **It's A Fact!!**
> In between periods, it is normal to have a clear or whitish fluid or discharge coming from your vagina. It should not itch or be uncomfortable. It should not smell bad.

Getting care on a regular basis is important. Your doctor will talk to you about how to take care of your changing body, how to tell if you have a vaginal infection, why abstinence is the healthiest choice, and how to protect yourself from sexually transmitted infections if you are sexually active. A doctor will also talk to you about your period and will help you out if you are having any problems.

How do I make an appointment?

Talk to your parent or guardian. Or, if you don't think you can talk to your parent or guardian, talk to someone else you trust about how to make an appointment. It is common to feel nervous about going to a clinic, especially when you're a teenager. But being scared is not a reason to skip out. Some of your friends may say they don't need to go, but it's the smart thing to do. A checkup is one important way to keep yourself healthy.

What happens at a visit?

Part of your first visit may be just to talk so you can get to know each other. Your doctor may ask a lot of questions about you and your family. You can also ask the doctor any questions you have. You don't have to be scared or embarrassed. Many teens have the same questions and concerns. You can also talk to your doctor about: cramps and problem periods; acne; weight issues; sexually transmitted infections; and having the blues or depression.

During your visit, your doctor will check your height, weight, and blood pressure. He or she may also do the following exams:

- **Breast Exam:** It is really common for young women to have some lumpiness in their breasts, but your doctor will check your breasts to make sure you don't have strange lumps or pain.

- **Pelvic Exam:** The doctor will examine inside your pelvic area to make sure your reproductive organs are healthy. The doctor will check out the outside of your genital area (the vulva) and will then use a tool called a speculum to look inside your vagina to see your cervix. Finally, the doctor will feel inside to make sure your internal organs feel okay. There will be pressure, but it should not be painful. Try to relax and breathe.

- **Pap Test:** If you are 21 or older or within three years of your first sexual experience, you should have a Pap test. This test is done to make sure the cells in your cervix are normal. The doctor will lightly swab your cervix during your pelvic exam to gather cells that can be looked at on a slide at a lab. It is best to have a Pap test when you don't have your period. If there are any problems with your cells, you will be contacted.

❖ It's A Fact!!

If you are sexually active, it is especially important to have a Pap test. The Pap test helps the doctor know if more tests are needed to see if you are infected with the human papillomavirus (HPV). Left untreated, this virus can lead to cervical cancer.

Doctors don't always test for STIs during your exam. If you're sexually active, ask to be tested for all STIs.

If it makes you more comfortable, you can have your mom, sister, or a friend stay in the room with you during the exam. If the doctor is male, a female nurse or assistant will also be in the room.

Chapter 19

Abnormal Pap Tests

What is a Pap test?

The Pap test, also called a Pap smear, checks for changes in the cells of your cervix. The cervix is the lower part of the uterus (womb) that opens into the vagina (birth canal). The Pap test can tell if you have an infection, abnormal (unhealthy) cervical cells, or cervical cancer.

Why do I need a Pap test?

A Pap test can save your life. It can find the earliest signs of cervical cancer. If cervical cancer is caught early, the chance of curing it is very high. Pap tests also can find infections and abnormal cervical cells that can turn into cancer cells. Treatment can prevent most cases of cervical cancer from developing.

Getting regular Pap tests is the best thing you can do to prevent cervical cancer. In fact, regular Pap tests have led to a major decline in the number of cervical cancer cases and deaths.

Do all women need Pap tests?

It is important for all women to have Pap tests, along with pelvic exams, as part of their routine health care. You need a Pap test if you are 21 years or older.

About This Chapter: Information in this chapter is from "Pap Test: Frequently Asked Questions," a publication of the U.S. Department of Health and Human Services, January 2010.

How often do I need to get a Pap test?

It depends on your age and health history. Talk with your doctor about what is best for you.

Who does not need regular Pap tests?

The only women who do not need regular Pap tests are:

- Women over age 65 who have had three normal Pap tests in a row and no abnormal test results in the last 10 years, and have been told by their doctors that they don't need to be tested anymore.

- Women who do not have a cervix and are at low risk for cervical cancer. These women should speak to their doctor before stopping regular Pap tests.

How can I reduce my chances of getting cervical cancer?

Aside from getting Pap tests, the best way to avoid cervical cancer is by steering clear of the human papillomavirus (HPV). HPV is a major cause of cervical cancer. HPV infection is also one of the most common sexually transmitted infections (STIs). So, a woman boosts her chances of getting cervical cancer if she: starts having sex before age 18; has many sex partners; has sex partners who have other sex partners; currently has a STI; or has ever had a STI.

What should I know about HPV?

Human papillomaviruses are a group of more than 100 different viruses.

- About 40 types of HPV are spread during sex.
- Some types of HPVs can cause cervical cancer when not treated.
- HPV infection is one of the most common STIs.
- About 75 percent of sexually active people will get HPV sometime in their life.
- Most women with untreated HPV do not get cervical cancer.
- Some HPVs cause genital warts but these HPVs do not cause cervical cancer.

- Since HPV rarely causes symptoms, most people don't know they have the infection.

How would I know if I had HPV?

Most women never know they have HPV. It usually stays hidden and doesn't cause symptoms like warts. When HPV doesn't go away on its own, it can cause changes in the cells of the cervix. Pap tests usually find these changes.

How do I prepare for a Pap test?

Many things can cause wrong test results by washing away or hiding abnormal cells of the cervix. So, doctors suggest that for two days before the test you avoid these practices:

- Douching
- Using tampons
- Using vaginal creams, suppositories, and medicines
- Using vaginal deodorant sprays or powders
- Having sex

Should I get a Pap test when I have my period?

No. Doctors suggest you schedule a Pap test when you do not have your period. The best time to be tested is 10 to 20 days after the first day of your last period.

How is a Pap test done?

Your doctor can do a Pap test during a pelvic exam. It is a simple and quick test. While you lie on an exam table, the doctor puts an instrument called a

---

❖ It's A Fact!!

Women who are living with human immunodeficiency virus (HIV), the virus that causes acquired immune deficiency syndrome (AIDS), are at a higher risk of cervical cancer and other cervical diseases. The U.S. Centers for Disease Control and Prevention recommends that all HIV-positive women get an initial Pap test, and get retested six months later. If both Pap tests are normal, then these women can get yearly Pap tests in the future.

speculum into your vagina, opening it to see the cervix. She will then use a special stick or brush to take a few cells from inside and around the cervix. The cells are placed on a glass slide and sent to a lab for examination. While usually painless, a Pap test is uncomfortable for some women.

When will I get the results of my Pap test?

Usually it takes three weeks to get Pap test results. Most of the time, test results are normal. If the test shows that something might be wrong, your doctor will contact you to schedule more tests. There are many reasons for abnormal Pap test results. It usually does not mean you have cancer.

What do abnormal Pap test results mean?

It is scary to hear that your Pap test results are abnormal. But abnormal Pap test results usually do not mean you have cancer. Most often there is a small problem with the cervix.

Some abnormal cells will turn into cancer. But most of the time, these unhealthy cells will go away on their own. Treating these unhealthy cells can prevent almost all cases of cervical cancer. If you have abnormal results, talk with your doctor about what they mean.

My Pap test was abnormal. What happens now?

There are many reasons for abnormal Pap test results. If results of the Pap test are unclear or show a small change in the cells of the cervix, your doctor will probably repeat the Pap test.

♣ It's A Fact!!

The Food and Drug Administration (FDA) recently approved a system that can help doctors see areas on the cervix that are likely to contain precancerous cells. The doctor uses this device right after a colposcopy. This system shines a light on the cervix and looks at how different areas of the cervix respond to this light. It gives a score to tiny areas of the cervix. It then makes a color map that helps the doctor decide where to further test the tissue with a biopsy. The colors and patterns on the map help the doctor tell between healthy tissue and tissue that might be diseased.

If the test finds more serious changes in the cells of the cervix, the doctor will suggest more powerful tests. Results of these tests will help your doctor decide on the best treatment. These include:

- **Colposcopy:** The doctor uses a tool called a colposcope to see the cells of the vagina and cervix in detail.

- **Endocervical Curettage:** The doctor takes a sample of cells from the endocervical canal with a small spoon-shaped tool called a curette.

- **Biopsy:** The doctor removes a small sample of cervical tissue. The sample is sent to a lab to be studied under a microscope.

My Pap test result was a false positive. What does this mean?

Pap tests are not always 100 percent correct. False positive and false negative results can happen. This can be upsetting and confusing. A false positive Pap test is when a woman is told she has abnormal cervical cells, but the cells are really normal. If your doctor says your Pap results were a false positive, there is no problem.

A false negative Pap test is when a woman is told her cells are normal, but in fact, there is a problem with the cervical cells that was missed. False negatives delay the discovery and treatment of unhealthy cells of the cervix. But, having regular Pap tests boosts your chances of finding any problems. If abnormal cells are missed at one time, they will probably be found on your next Pap test.

I don't have health insurance. How can I get a free or low-cost Pap test?

Programs funded by the National Breast and Cervical Cancer Early Detection Program (NBCCEDP) offer free or low-cost Pap tests to women in need. These and other programs are available throughout the United States. Your state or local health department can direct you to places that offer free or low-cost Pap tests.

Chapter 20

Getting The HPV Vaccine

Why are human papillomavirus (HPV) vaccines needed?

HPV vaccines prevent serious health problems such as cervical cancer and other, less common cancers which are caused by HPV. In addition to cancer, HPV can also cause other health problems, such as genital warts. HPV is a common virus that is easily spread by skin-to-skin contact during sexual activity with another person. It is possible to have HPV without knowing it, so it is possible to unknowingly spread HPV to another person. Safe, effective vaccines are available to protect females and males against some of the most common types of HPV and the health problems that the virus can cause.

How common are the health problems caused by HPV?

HPV is the main cause of cervical cancer in women. There are about 11,000 new cervical cancer cases each year in the United States. Cervical cancer causes about 4,000 deaths in women each year in the United States.

What HPV vaccines are available in the United States?

Two HPV vaccines are licensed by the Food and Drug Administration (FDA) and recommended by the Centers for Disease Control and Prevention

About This Chapter: Information in this chapter is from "HPV Vaccine—Questions and Answers," a publication of the Centers for Disease Control and Prevention, December 2009. Reviewed January 2010.

(CDC). These vaccines are Cervarix (made by GlaxoSmithKline) and Gardasil (made by Merck).

How are the two HPV vaccines similar?

- Both vaccines are very effective against HPV types 16 and 18, which cause most cervical cancers. So both vaccines prevent cervical cancer and precancer in women.

> ✤ **It's A Fact!!**
> About one in 100 sexually active adults in the United States have genital warts at any one time.

- Both vaccines are very safe.

- Both vaccines are made with very small parts of HPV that cannot cause infection with HPV, so neither of the vaccines can cause HPV infection.

- Both vaccines are given as shots and require three doses.

How are the two HPV vaccines different?

- Only one of the vaccines (Gardasil) also protects against HPV types 6 and 11. These HPV types cause most genital warts in females and males.

- The vaccines have different adjuvants—a vaccine adjuvant is a substance that is added to the vaccine to increase the body's immune response.

Who should get HPV vaccine?

Cervarix and Gardasil are licensed, safe, and effective for females ages nine through 26 years. CDC recommends that all girls who are 11 or 12 years old get the three doses (shots) of either brand of HPV vaccine to protect against cervical cancer and precancer. Gardasil also protects against most genital warts. Girls and young women ages 13 through 26 should get all three doses of an HPV vaccine if they have not received all doses yet.

People who have already had sexual contact before getting all three doses of an HPV vaccine might still benefit if they were not infected before vaccination with the HPV types included in the vaccine they received. The best way to be sure that a person gets the most benefit from HPV vaccination is to complete all three doses before sexual activity begins.

Why is HPV vaccine recommended at ages 11 or 12 years?

For the HPV vaccine to work best, it is very important to get all three doses (shots) before being exposed to HPV. Someone can be infected with HPV the very first time they have sexual contact with another person. It is also possible to get HPV even if sexual contact only happens one time.

How does getting HPV vaccine at ages 11 or 12 fit with other health recommendations?

Doctors recommend health checkups for preteens. The first dose of an HPV vaccine should be given to girls aged 11 or 12 years during a preteen health checkup. The first dose of Gardasil can also be given to boys during their preteen checkups. Two other vaccines are recommended for preteens. During one visit, either HPV vaccine can be given safely with these other preteen vaccines. A checkup in the preteen years is also a time when preteens and their parents can talk to their providers about other ways to stay healthy and safe.

What is the recommended schedule (or timing) of the three HPV doses (shots)?

For both females and males, three doses (shots) are needed. CDC recommends that the second dose be given one to two months after the first, and the third dose be given six months after the first dose.

Will someone be protected against HPV-related diseases if they do not get all three doses?

No studies so far have shown whether or not one or two doses protect as well as getting three doses, so it is very important to get all three doses.

✤ It's A Fact!!

Gardasil is also licensed, safe, and effective for males ages nine through 26 years. Boys and young men may choose to get this vaccine to prevent genital warts.

Are the HPV vaccines safe and effective?

FDA has licensed the vaccines as safe and effective. Both vaccines were tested in thousands of people around the world. These studies showed no serious side effects. Common, mild side effects included pain where the shot was given, fever, headache, and nausea. As with all vaccines, CDC and FDA continue to monitor the safety of these vaccines very carefully.

Do people faint after getting HPV vaccines?

People faint for many reasons. Some people may faint after getting any vaccine, including HPV vaccines. Falls and injuries can occur after fainting. Sitting or lying down for about 15 minutes after a vaccination can help prevent fainting and injuries.

Can HPV vaccines treat HPV infections, cancers, or warts?

HPV vaccines will not treat or get rid of existing HPV infections. Also, HPV vaccines do not treat or cure health problems (like cancer or warts) caused by an HPV infection that occurred before vaccination.

Are there other HPV diseases that the two vaccines may prevent?

Studies have shown that Gardasil prevents cancers of the vagina and vulva, which can be caused by HPV types 16 and 18. Studies of Cervarix have not specifically looked at protection against vaginal and vulvar cancers.

Published studies have not looked at other health problems that might be prevented by HPV vaccines. It is possible that HPV vaccines will also prevent cancers of the head and neck, penis, and anus due to HPV 16 or 18. Gardasil might prevent recurrent respiratory papillomatosis (RRP), a rare condition caused by HPV 6 or 11 in which warts grow in the throat.

Are kids getting too many vaccines?

Vaccines strengthen the body's immune system—they do not overload it. No reputable science shows that getting recommended vaccines hurts the immune systems of healthy kids. The HPV vaccines are important tools to prevent cervical cancer and genital warts. As with all vaccines, the benefits outweigh potential risks.

Why aren't HPV vaccines recommended for people older than 26?

Both vaccines were studied in thousands of people from nine through 26 years old and found to be safe and effective for these ages. The FDA will consider licensing HPV vaccines for other ages if new studies show that this would also be safe and effective.

Should pregnant women be vaccinated?

Pregnant women are not included in the recommendations for HPV vaccines. Studies show neither vaccine caused problems for babies born to women who got the HPV vaccine while they were pregnant. Getting the HPV vaccine when pregnant is not a reason to consider ending a pregnancy. But, to be on the safe side until even more is known, a pregnant woman should not get any doses of either HPV vaccine until her pregnancy is completed.

What should a woman do if she realizes she received HPV vaccination while pregnant?

If a woman realizes that she got any shots of an HPV vaccine while pregnant, she should do two things:

- Wait until after her pregnancy to finish the remaining HPV vaccine doses.

- Report the vaccination to the appropriate pregnancy registry. There are pregnancy registries to help us learn more about how pregnant women respond to each of the vaccines. So, if a woman realizes that she got any shots of either HPV vaccine while pregnant, she should work with her health care provider to report it to the appropriate pregnancy registry.

Will HPV vaccination be covered by health insurance?

Most health insurance plans cover recommended vaccines. But there may be a lag time after a vaccine is recommended before it gets added to insurance plans. Some insurance plans may not cover any or all vaccines. Check with your insurance provider to see if the cost of the vaccine is covered before going to the doctor.

Chapter 21

Douching

What is douching?

The word douche means to wash or soak in French. Douching is washing or cleaning out the vagina (birth canal) with water or other mixtures of fluids. Most douches are prepackaged mixes of water and vinegar, baking soda, or iodine. You can buy these products at drug and grocery stores. The mixtures usually come in a bottle and can be squirted into the vagina through a tube or nozzle.

Why do women douche?

Women douche because they mistakenly believe it gives many benefits. Women who douche say they do it for these reasons:

- Clean the vagina

- Rinse away blood after monthly periods

- Get rid of odor

- Avoid sexually transmitted infections (STIs)

- Prevent pregnancy

About This Chapter: Information in this chapter is from "Douching: Frequently Asked Questions," a publication of the U.S. Department of Health and Human Services, May 2010.

How common is douching?

Douching is common among women in the United States. It's estimated that 20 to 40 percent of American women 15 to 44 years old douche regularly. About half of these women douche each week. Higher rates of douching are seen in teens, African-American women, and Hispanic women.

Is douching safe?

Most doctors and the American Congress of Obstetricians and Gynecologists (ACOG) recommend that women don't douche. Douching can change the delicate balance of vaginal flora (organisms that live in the vagina) and acidity in a healthy vagina. One way to look at it is in a healthy vagina there are both good and bad bacteria. The balance of the good and bad bacteria help maintain an acidic environment. Any changes can cause an overgrowth of bad bacteria which can lead to a yeast infection or bacterial vaginosis. Plus, if you have a vaginal infection, douching can push the bacteria causing the infection up into the uterus, fallopian tubes, and ovaries.

What are the dangers linked to douching?

Research shows that women who douche regularly have more health problems than women who don't. Doctors are still unsure whether douching causes these problems. Douching may simply be more common in groups of women who tend to have these issues. Health problems linked to douching include the following:

- Vaginal irritation
- Bacterial vaginosis (BV)
- STIs
- Pelvic inflammatory disease (PID)

❧ It's A Fact!!

Some sexually transmitted infections (STIs), bacterial vaginosis, and pelvic inflammatory disease can all lead to serious problems during pregnancy. These include infection in the baby, problems with labor, and early delivery.

Should I douche to clean inside my vagina?

No. The ACOG suggests women avoid douching completely. In most cases the vagina's acidic environment cleans the vagina. If there is a strong odor or irritation it usually means something is wrong. Douching can increase your chances of infection. The only time you should douche is when your doctor tells you to.

What is the best way to clean my vagina?

Most doctors say it's best to let your vagina clean itself. The vagina cleans itself naturally by making mucous. The mucous washes away blood, semen, and vaginal discharge. You should know that even healthy, clean vaginas may have a mild odor.

Keep the outside of your vagina clean and healthy by washing regularly with warm water and mild soap when you bathe. You should also avoid scented tampons, pads, powders, and sprays. These products may increase your chances of getting a vaginal infection.

Should I douche to get rid of vaginal odor, discharge, pain, itching, or burning?

No. You should never douche to try to get rid of vaginal odor, discharge, pain, itching, or burning. Douching will only cover up odor and make other problems worse. It's very important to call your doctor right away if you have symptoms such as these:

- Vaginal discharge that smells bad
- Thick, white, or yellowish-green discharge with or without an odor
- Burning, redness, and swelling in or around the vagina
- Pain when urinating
- Pain or discomfort during sex

These may be signs of an infection, especially one that may be sexually transmitted. Do not douche before seeing your doctor. This can make it hard for the doctor to figure out what's wrong.

Can douching after sex prevent STIs?

No. It's a myth that douching after sex can prevent STIs. The only sure way to prevent STIs is to not have sex. If you do have sex, the best way to prevent STIs is to practice safer sex:

• Be faithful. Have sex with only one partner who has been tested for STIs and is not infected.

• Use latex or female condoms every time you have sex.

• Avoid contact with semen, blood, vaginal fluids, and sores on your partner's genitals.

Can douching after sex stop me from getting pregnant?

No. Douching does not prevent pregnancy. It should never be used for birth control.

Can douching hurt my chances of having a healthy pregnancy?

Douching may affect your chances of having a healthy pregnancy. Limited research shows that douching may make it harder for you to get pregnant. In women trying to get pregnant, those who douched more than once a week took the longest to get pregnant.

✤ It's A Fact!!
Studies also show that douching may increase a woman's chance of damaged fallopian tubes and ectopic pregnancy. Ectopic pregnancy is when the fertilized egg attaches to the inside of the fallopian tube instead of the uterus. If left untreated, ectopic pregnancy can be life threatening. It can also make it hard for a woman to get pregnant in the future.

Chapter 22

Medical Uses For Oral Contraceptives

Adolescent girls and young women are frequently prescribed oral contraceptive pills for irregular or absent menstrual periods, menstrual cramps, acne, premenstrual syndrome (PMS), polycystic ovary syndrome (PCOS), endometriosis, and hormone replacement therapy.

What Are Oral Contraceptive Pills?

Oral contraceptive pills (also called the "Pill," OCPs, or hormonal pills) contain two types of synthetic (man-made) female hormones: progestin and estrogen. These hormones are normally made by the ovaries. There are many different types of oral contraceptives.

What Kinds Of Medical Conditions Can Be Helped With The Oral Contraceptive Pills?

Polycystic Ovary Syndrome (PCOS): A hormone imbalance which causes irregular menstrual periods, acne, and excess hair growth. Oral contraceptive pills work by lowering certain hormone levels to regulate menstrual periods. When hormone levels are back to normal, acne and hair growth often improve.

About This Chapter: Information in this chapter is from "Medical Uses of the Oral Contraceptive Pill: A Guide for Teens, " Copyright © 2010 Center for Young Women's Health, Children's Hospital Boston. All rights reserved. Used with permission. www .youngwomenshealth.org.

Endometriosis: Most girls with endometriosis have cramps or pelvic pain during their menstrual cycle. Oral contraceptive pills are often prescribed to treat endometriosis and work by temporarily turning off the ovaries so ovulation does not happen. When hormonal treatment is prescribed continuously, young women will rarely have periods, or not at all. Since periods can cause pain for young women with endometriosis, stopping periods will usually improve cramps and pelvic pain.

Lack Of Periods ("Amenorrhea") From Low Weight, Stress, Excessive Exercise, Or Damage To The Ovaries From Radiation Or Chemotherapy: With any of these conditions, the hormone "estrogen" is not made in normal amounts by the body. Oral contraceptive pills may be prescribed to replace estrogen, which helps to regulate the menstrual cycle. For girls whose menstrual periods are irregular (too few—or not at all), oral contraceptive pills can help to regulate the menstrual cycle to every 28 days and provide the body with normal amounts of estrogen to keep bones healthy.

Menstrual Cramps: When over-the-counter medications don't help with severe cramps, oral contraceptive pills may be the solution because they prevent ovulation and lighten periods.

Premenstrual Syndrome (PMS): Symptoms of PMS such as mood swings, breast soreness, bloating, and acne can occur up to two weeks before a young woman's period. Oral contraceptives pills are often prescribed to stop ovulation and keep hormone levels even. Symptoms usually improve, particularly when the OCPs are prescribed continuously.

Heavy Menstrual Periods: Oral contraceptive pills can reduce the amount and length of menstrual bleeding.

Acne: For moderate to severe acne, which over-the-counter and prescription medications can't cure, oral contraceptive

> ### ✤ It's A Fact!!
>
> - Besides birth control, there are many medical benefits of oral contraceptive pills (OCPs).
>
> - As with any medicine there are possible side effects and risks.
>
> - OCPs can help irregular periods, PCOS, endometriosis, acne, menstrual cramps, and low estrogen conditions.

pills may be prescribed. The hormones in the oral contraceptive pill can help stop acne from forming. Be patient though, since it takes several months for the oral contraceptive pills to work.

Other Medical Benefits

Because there is less menstrual bleeding with the use of oral contraceptive pills, you are less likely to get anemia (low number of red blood cells, which carry oxygen from the lungs to the tissues). Oral contraceptive pills decrease your chance of getting endometrial (lining of the uterus) cancer, ovarian cancer, and ovarian cysts.

Are There Side Effects From Taking The Oral Contraceptive Pill?

Most women have no side effects when taking the oral contraceptive pill, but some women do experience irregular periods, nausea, headaches, or weight change. Each type of oral contraceptive pill can affect each woman differently.

Spotting between periods may occur during the first three weeks of taking hormone pills, and can continue for up to three cycles, but this is not serious. You should call your health care provider if the bleeding is heavier than a light flow, or lasts more than a few days.

Some women have nausea, but this usually goes away if the Pill is taken with a meal or a snack at bedtime. Sometimes a pill with less estrogen is prescribed if the nausea doesn't go away.

Sometimes, women may experience headaches when they start taking oral contraceptive pills, but headaches usually happen because of stress or other reasons. If your health care provider thinks they are related to the Pill, he/she may prescribe an oral contraceptive pill with a lower dose of estrogen or may sometimes take you off the oral contraceptive pill.

Mood changes can occur while taking the oral contraceptive pill. Exercise and a healthy diet may help, but if they don't, you may need to talk to your health care provider and try a different kind of oral contraceptive pill. Your breasts may become tender or may get larger. Your appetite may increase, and a few teens feel bloated.

Some teens gain weight, some lose weight, but most teens stay exactly the same when they are taking the oral contraceptive pill. Many times a young woman thinks she has gained 5–10 pounds, but when her weight is actually measured, there is no change. If you think you may have gained weight due to the Pill, you should see your health care provider and get your weight checked. If you do gain weight, or you want to prevent gaining weight, you should make sure that you eat a healthy diet. Eat plenty of fruits and vegetables every day, avoid fast food, and get enough exercise! If these ideas don't help, talk to your health care provider.

Are There Any Risks If I Take The Oral Contraceptive Pill?

Oral contraceptive pills with estrogen may cause a slight increase in the risk of developing blood clots in the legs. Among women who do not take the Pill, five out of 100,000 women per year develop blood clots. Among women who do take the Pill, the risk slightly increases to 15–20 out of 100,000 women per year. Find out if anyone in your family (blood relative) has had blood clots, especially when they were young. And if you are a smoker, try to quit as soon as possible.

Chapter 23

Vaginal Infections

What is a vaginal yeast infection?

A vaginal yeast infection is irritation of the vagina and the area around it called the vulva. Yeast is a type of fungus. Yeast infections are caused by overgrowth of the fungus *Candida albicans*. Small amounts of yeast are always in the vagina. But when too much yeast grows, you can get an infection. Yeast infections are very common. About 75 percent of women have one during their lives. And almost half of women have two or more vaginal yeast infections.

What are the signs of a vaginal yeast infection?

The most common symptom of a yeast infection is extreme itchiness in and around the vagina. Other symptoms include: burning, redness, and swelling of the vagina and the vulva; pain when passing urine and/or during sex; soreness; a thick, white vaginal discharge that looks like cottage cheese and does not have a bad smell; and a rash on the vagina.

About This Chapter: Information in this chapter is from the following publications of the U.S. Department of Health and Human Services: "Vaginal Yeast Infections: Frequently Asked Questions," September 2008; "Urinary Tract Infection: Frequently Asked Questions," May 2008; and "Bacterial Vaginosis: Frequently Asked Questions," September 2008.

Should I call my doctor if I think I have a yeast infection?

Yes, you need to see your doctor to find out for sure if you have a yeast infection. The signs of a yeast infection are much like those of sexually transmitted infections (STIs) like chlamydia and gonorrhea. So, it's hard to be sure you have a yeast infection and not something more serious.

How is a vaginal yeast infection diagnosed?

Your doctor will do a pelvic exam to look for swelling and discharge. Your doctor may also use a swab to take a fluid sample from your vagina. A quick look with a microscope or a lab test will show if yeast is causing the problem.

Why did I get a yeast infection?

Many things can raise your risk of a vaginal yeast infection, such as: stress; lack of sleep; illness; poor eating habits, including eating extreme amounts of sugary foods; pregnancy; having your period; taking certain medicines, including birth control pills, antibiotics, and steroids; diseases such as poorly controlled diabetes and human immunodeficiency virus (HIV)/acquired immune deficiency syndrome (AIDS); and hormonal changes during your periods.

Can I get a yeast infection from having sex?

Yes, but it is rare. Most often, women don't get yeast infections from sex. The most common cause is a weak immune system.

✔ Quick Tip

If you keep getting yeast infections, be sure and talk with your doctor. About five percent of women get four or more vaginal yeast infections in one year. This is called recurrent vulvovaginal candidiasis (RVVC). RVVC is more common in women with diabetes or weak immune systems. Doctors most often treat this problem with antifungal medicine for up to six months.

Source: "Vaginal Yeast Infections," U.S. Department of Health and Human Services, September 2008.

How are yeast infections treated?

Yeast infections can be cured with antifungal medicines that come as creams, tablets, and ointments or suppositories that are inserted into the vagina. These products can be bought over the counter at the drug store or grocery store. Your doctor can also prescribe you a single dose of oral fluconazole. But do not use this drug if you are pregnant.

Is it safe to use over-the-counter medicines for yeast infections?

Yes, but always talk with your doctor before treating yourself for a vaginal yeast infection if you are pregnant, have never been diagnosed with a yeast infection, or keep getting yeast infections.

If I have a yeast infection, does my sexual partner need to be treated?

Yeast infections are not STIs, and health experts don't know for sure if they are transmitted sexually. About 12 to 15 percent of men get an itchy rash on the penis if they have unprotected sex with an infected woman. If this happens to your partner, he should see a doctor. Men who haven't been circumcised are at higher risk. Lesbians may be at risk for spreading yeast infections to their partner(s). Research is still being done to find out. If your female partner has any symptoms, she should also be tested and treated.

How can I avoid getting another yeast infection?

To prevent yeast infections, avoid douches; scented hygiene products like bubble bath, sprays, pads, and tampons; hot tubs and very hot baths; and tight underwear or clothes made of synthetic fibers. You should also: change tampons and pads often during your period; wear cotton underwear and pantyhose with a cotton crotch; and change out of wet swimsuits and exercise clothes as soon as you can.

What is a urinary tract infection (UTI)?

A UTI is an infection anywhere in the urinary tract. The urinary tract makes and stores urine and removes it from the body.

What causes UTIs?

Bacteria, a type of germ that gets into your urinary tract, cause a UTI. This can happen in many ways:

- Wiping from back to front after a bowel movement (BM)(germs can get into your urethra, which has its opening in front of the vagina)

- Having sexual intercourse (germs in the vagina can be pushed into the urethra)

- Waiting too long to pass urine

- Using a diaphragm for birth control, or spermicides (creams that kill sperm) with a diaphragm or on a condom

- Anything that makes it hard to completely empty your bladder, like a kidney stone

- Having diabetes, which makes it harder for your body to fight other health problems

- Loss of estrogen (a hormone) and changes in the vagina after menopause

- Having had a catheter in place

What are the signs of a UTI?

The signs of a UTI include: pain or stinging when you pass urine; an urge to pass urine a lot, but not much comes out when you go; pressure in your lower belly; urine that smells bad or looks milky, cloudy, or reddish in color; and feeling tired or shaky or having a fever.

✎ What's It Mean?

Catheter: A catheter is a thin tube put through the urethra into the bladder. It's used to drain urine during a medical test and for people who cannot pass urine on their own.

Source: U.S. Department of Health and Human Services, May 2008.

How does a doctor find out if I have a UTI?

To find out if you have a UTI, your doctor will need to test a clean sample of your urine. If you are prone to UTIs, your doctor may want to take pictures of your urinary tract with an x-ray or ultrasound. These pictures can show swelling, stones, or blockage. Your doctor also may want to look inside your bladder using a cystoscope, which is a small tube that's put into the urethra to see inside of the urethra and bladder.

✔ **Quick Tip**

If you see blood in your urine, tell a doctor right away.

Source: U.S. Department of Health and Human Services, May 2008.

How is a UTI treated?

UTIs are treated with antibiotics, medicines that kill the bacteria that cause the infection. Your doctor will tell you how long you need to take the medicine. Make sure you take all of your medicine, even if you feel better. Many women feel better in one or two days.

Will a UTI hurt my kidneys?

If treated right away, a UTI is not likely to damage your kidneys or urinary tract. But UTIs that are not treated can cause serious problems in your kidneys and the rest of your body.

How can I keep from getting UTIs?

These are steps you can take to try to prevent a UTI. But you may follow these steps and still get a UTI. If you have symptoms of a UTI, call your doctor.

- Urinate when you need to. Don't hold it. Pass urine before and after sex. After you pass urine or have a bowel movement, wipe from front to back.

- Drink water every day and after sex.

- Clean the outer lips of your vagina and anus each day.

- Don't use douches or feminine hygiene sprays.

- If you get a lot of UTIs and use spermicides, or creams that kill sperm, talk to your doctor about using other forms of birth control.

- Wear underpants with a cotton crotch. Don't wear tight-fitting pants, which can trap in moisture.

- Take showers instead of tub baths.

What is bacterial vaginosis (BV)?

The vagina normally has a balance of mostly good bacteria and fewer harmful bacteria. Bacterial vaginosis, known as BV, develops when the balance changes. With BV, there is an increase in harmful bacteria and a decrease in good bacteria. BV is the most common vaginal infection in women of childbearing age.

> ♣ **It's A Fact!!**
> If you don't take medicine for a UTI, the UTI can hurt other parts of your body. Also, if you're pregnant and have signs of a UTI, see your doctor right away. A UTI could cause problems in your pregnancy, such as having your baby too early or getting high blood pressure. Also, UTIs in pregnant women are more likely to travel to the kidneys.
>
> Source: U.S. Department of Health and Human Services, May 2008.

What causes BV?

Not much is known about how women get BV. Any woman can get BV. But there are certain things that can upset the normal balance of bacteria in the vagina, raising your risk of BV:

- Having a new sex partner or multiple sex partners

- Douching

- Using an intrauterine device (IUD) for birth control

- Not using a condom

> ♣ **It's A Fact!!**
> BV is more common among women who are sexually active, but it is not clear how sex changes the balance of bacteria.
>
> Source: "Bacterial Vaginosis," U.S. Department of Health and Human Services, September 2008.

What are the signs of BV?

Women with BV may have an abnormal vaginal discharge with an unpleasant odor. Some women report a strong fish-like odor, especially after sex. The discharge can be white (milky) or gray. It may also be foamy or watery. Other symptoms may include burning when urinating, itching around the outside of the vagina, and irritation. These symptoms may also be caused by another type of infection, so it is important to see a doctor. Some women with BV have no symptoms at all.

How can I find out if I have BV?

There is a test to find out if you have BV. Your doctor takes a sample of fluid from your vagina and has it tested. Your doctor may also see signs of BV during an examination of the vagina.

How is BV treated?

BV is treated with antibiotic medicines prescribed by your doctor. Your doctor may give you either metronidazole or clindamycin.

✤ It's A Fact!!

Generally, male sex partners of women with BV don't need to be treated. However, BV can be spread to female partners. If your current partner is female, talk to her about treatment. You can get BV again even after being treated.

Source: "Bacterial Vaginosis," U.S. Department of Health and Human Services, September 2008.

Chapter 24

Pelvic Inflammatory Disease

What is PID?

Pelvic inflammatory disease (PID) refers to infection of the uterus (womb), fallopian tubes (tubes that carry eggs from the ovaries to the uterus), and other reproductive organs that causes symptoms such as lower abdominal pain. It is a serious complication of some sexually transmitted diseases (STDs), especially chlamydia and gonorrhea. PID can damage the fallopian tubes and tissues in and near the uterus and ovaries. PID can lead to serious consequences including infertility, ectopic pregnancy (a pregnancy in the fallopian tube or elsewhere outside of the womb), abscess formation, and chronic pelvic pain.

How common is PID?

Each year in the United States, it is estimated that more than 750,000 women experience an episode of acute PID. More than 75,000 women may become infertile each year as a result of PID, and a large proportion of the ectopic pregnancies occurring every year are due to the consequences of PID.

How do women get PID?

PID occurs when bacteria move upward from a woman's vagina or cervix (opening to the uterus) into her reproductive organs. Many different organisms

About This Chapter: Information in this chapter is from "PID (Pelvic Inflammatory Disease)," a fact sheet from the Centers for Disease Control and Prevention, May 2010.

can cause PID, but many cases are associated with gonorrhea and chlamydia, two very common bacterial STDs. A prior episode of PID increases the risk of another episode because the reproductive organs may be damaged during the initial bout of infection.

The more sex partners a woman has, the greater her risk of developing PID. Also, a woman whose partner has more than one sex partner is at greater risk of developing PID, because of the potential for more exposure to infectious agents.

Women who douche may have a higher risk of developing PID compared with women who do not douche. Research has shown that douching changes the vaginal flora (organisms that live in the vagina) in harmful ways, and can force bacteria into the upper reproductive organs from the vagina.

Women who have an intrauterine device (IUD) inserted may have a slightly increased risk of PID near the time of insertion compared with women using other contraceptives or no contraceptive at all. However, this risk is greatly reduced if a woman is tested and, if necessary, treated for STDs before an IUD is inserted.

What are the signs and symptoms?

Symptoms of PID vary from mild to severe. When PID is caused by chlamydial infection, a woman may be more likely to experience mild symptoms or no symptoms at all, while serious damage is being done to her reproductive organs. Chlamydia can also cause fallopian tube infection without any symptoms. Because of vague symptoms, PID often goes unrecognized by women and their health care providers. Women who have symptoms of PID most commonly have lower abdominal pain. Other signs and symptoms include fever, unusual vaginal discharge that may have a foul odor, painful intercourse, painful urination, irregular menstrual bleeding, and pain in the right upper abdomen (rare).

What are the complications of PID?

Prompt and appropriate treatment can help prevent complications of PID, including permanent damage to the female reproductive organs. Infection-causing bacteria can invade the fallopian tubes, causing normal tissue to turn into scar tissue. This scar tissue blocks or interrupts the normal movement of eggs into the uterus. If the fallopian tubes are totally blocked by scar tissue, sperm cannot fertilize an egg, and the woman becomes infertile. Infertility also can occur if the fallopian tubes are partially blocked or even slightly damaged.

About one in ten women with PID becomes infertile, and if a woman has multiple episodes of PID, her chances of becoming infertile increase. In addition, a partially blocked or slightly damaged fallopian tube may cause a fertilized egg to remain in the fallopian tube. If this fertilized egg begins to grow in the tube as if it were in the uterus, it is called an ectopic pregnancy. As it grows, an ectopic pregnancy can rupture the fallopian tube causing severe pain, internal bleeding, and even death.

Scarring in the fallopian tubes and other pelvic structures can also cause chronic pelvic pain (pain that lasts for months or even years).

How is PID diagnosed?

PID is difficult to diagnose because the symptoms are often subtle and mild. Many episodes of PID go undetected because the woman or her health care provider fails to recognize the implications of mild or nonspecific symptoms. Because there are no precise tests for PID, a diagnosis is usually based on clinical findings. If symptoms such as lower abdominal pain are present, a health care provider should perform a physical examination to determine the nature and location of the pain and check for fever, abnormal vaginal or cervical discharge, and for evidence of gonorrheal or chlamydial infection. If the findings suggest PID, treatment is necessary.

❖ It's A Fact!!
Women with repeated episodes of PID are more likely to suffer infertility, ectopic pregnancy, or chronic pelvic pain.

The health care provider may also order tests to identify the infection-causing organism (e.g., chlamydial or gonorrheal infection) or to distinguish between PID and other problems with similar symptoms. A pelvic ultrasound is a helpful procedure for diagnosing PID. An ultrasound can view the pelvic area to see whether the fallopian tubes are enlarged or whether an abscess is present. In some cases, a laparoscopy may be necessary to confirm the diagnosis. A laparoscopy is a surgical procedure in which a thin, rigid tube with a lighted end and camera (laparoscope) is inserted through a small incision in the abdomen. This procedure enables the doctor to view the internal pelvic organs and to take specimens for laboratory studies, if needed.

> ✤ **It's A Fact!!**
> The longer a woman delays treatment for PID, the more likely she is to become infertile or to have a future ectopic pregnancy because of damage to the fallopian tubes.

What is the treatment for PID?

PID can be cured with several types of antibiotics. A health care provider will determine and prescribe the best therapy. However, antibiotic treatment does not reverse any damage that has already occurred to the reproductive organs. If a woman has pelvic pain and other symptoms of PID, it is critical that she seek care immediately. Prompt antibiotic treatment can prevent severe damage to reproductive organs.

Because of the difficulty in identifying organisms infecting the internal reproductive organs and because more than one organism may be responsible for an episode of PID, PID is usually treated with at least two antibiotics that are effective against a wide range of infectious agents. These antibiotics can be given by mouth or by injection. The symptoms may go away before the infection is cured. Even if symptoms go away, the woman should finish taking all of the prescribed medicine. This will help prevent the infection from returning. Women being treated for PID should be reevaluated by their health care provider two to three days after starting treatment to be sure the antibiotics are working to cure the infection. In addition, a woman's sex partner(s) should be treated to decrease the risk of reinfection. Although sex partners may have no symptoms, they may still be infected with the organisms that can cause PID.

Hospitalization to treat PID may be recommended if the woman has any of these characteristics:

- Is severely ill (e.g., nausea, vomiting, and high fever)

- Is pregnant

- Does not respond to or cannot take oral medication and needs intravenous antibiotics

- Has an abscess in the fallopian tube or ovary (tubo-ovarian abscess)

- Needs to be monitored to be sure that her symptoms are not due to another condition that would require emergency surgery (for example, appendicitis).

How can PID be prevented?

Women can protect themselves from PID by taking action to prevent STDs or by getting early treatment if they do get an STD. The surest way to avoid transmission of STDs is to abstain from sexual intercourse, or to be in a long-term mutually monogamous relationship with a partner who has been tested and is known to be uninfected.

Latex male condoms, when used consistently and correctly, can reduce the risk of transmission of chlamydia and gonorrhea. The Centers for Disease Control and Prevention (CDC) recommends yearly chlamydia testing of all sexually active women age 25 or younger, older women with risk factors for chlamydial infections (those who have a new sex partner or multiple sex partners), and all pregnant women. An appropriate sexual risk assessment by a health care provider should always be conducted and may indicate more frequent screening for some women.

❖ It's A Fact!!

If symptoms continue or if an abscess does not go away, surgery may be needed. Complications of PID, such as chronic pelvic pain and scarring, are difficult to treat, but sometimes they improve with surgery.

Any genital symptoms such as an unusual sore, discharge with odor, burning during urination, or bleeding between menstrual cycles could mean an STD infection. If a woman has any of these symptoms, she should stop having sex and consult a health care provider immediately. Treating STDs early can prevent PID. Women who are told they have an STD and are treated for it should notify all of their recent sex partners so they can see a health care provider and be evaluated for STDs. Sexual activity should not resume until all sex partners have been examined and, if necessary, treated.

Chapter 25

Ovarian Cysts

What are ovaries?

The ovaries are a pair of organs in the female reproductive system. They are located in the pelvis, one on each side of the uterus. The uterus is the hollow, pear-shaped organ where a baby grows. Each ovary is about the size and shape of an almond. The ovaries produce eggs and female hormones. Hormones are chemicals that control the way certain cells or organs function.

Every month, during a woman's menstrual cycle, an egg grows inside an ovary. It grows in a tiny sac called a follicle. When an egg matures, the sac breaks open to release the egg. The egg travels through the fallopian tube to the uterus for fertilization. Then the sac dissolves. The empty sac becomes corpus luteum. Corpus luteum makes hormones that help prepare for the next egg.

The ovaries are the main source of the female hormones estrogen and progesterone. These hormones affect many bodily functions including the following:

• The way breasts and body hair grow

• Body shape

• The menstrual cycle

• Pregnancy

About This Chapter: Information in this chapter is from "Ovarian Cysts: Frequently Asked Questions," a publication of the U.S. Department of Health and Human Services, September 2008.

What are ovarian cysts?

A cyst is a fluid-filled sac. Cysts can form anywhere in the body. Ovarian cysts form in or on the ovaries. The most common type of ovarian cyst is a functional cyst.

Functional cysts often form during the menstrual cycle. There are two types:

- **Follicle Cysts:** These cysts form when the sac doesn't break open to release the egg. Then the sac keeps growing. This type of cyst most often goes away in one to three months.

- **Corpus Luteum Cysts:** These cysts form if the sac doesn't dissolve. Instead, the sac seals off after the egg is released. Then fluid builds up inside. Most of these cysts go away after a few weeks. They can grow to almost four inches. They may bleed or twist the ovary and cause pain. They are rarely cancerous. Some drugs used to cause ovulation, such as Clomid® or Serophene®, can raise the risk of getting these cysts.

Other types of ovarian cysts include the following:

- **Endometriomas:** These cysts form in women who have endometriosis. This problem occurs when tissue that looks and acts like the lining of the uterus grows outside the uterus. The tissue may attach to the ovary and form a growth. These cysts can be painful during sex and during your period.

- **Cystadenomas:** These cysts form from cells on the outer surface of the ovary. They are often filled with a watery fluid or thick, sticky gel. They can become large and cause pain.

- **Dermoid Cysts:** These cysts contain many types of cells. They may be filled with hair, teeth, and other tissues that become part of the cyst. They can become large and cause pain.

- **Polycystic Ovaries:** These cysts are caused when eggs mature within the sacs but are not released. The cycle then repeats. The sacs continue to grow and many cysts form. For more information about polycystic ovaries, refer to the chapter about Polycystic Ovary Syndrome.

What are the symptoms of ovarian cysts?

Many ovarian cysts don't cause symptoms. Others can cause the following:

✔ **Quick Tip**

If you have these symptoms, get help right away:

- Pain with fever and vomiting

- Sudden, severe abdominal pain

- Faintness, dizziness, or weakness

- Rapid breathing

- Pressure, swelling, or pain in the abdomen

- Pelvic pain

- Dull ache in the lower back and thighs

- Problems passing urine completely

- Pain during sex

- Weight gain

- Pain during your period

- Abnormal bleeding

- Nausea or vomiting

- Breast tenderness

How are ovarian cysts found?

Doctors most often find ovarian cysts during routine pelvic exams. The doctor may feel the swelling of a cyst on the ovary. Once a cyst is found, tests are done to help plan treatment. Tests include the following:

- **An Ultrasound:** This test uses sound waves to create images of the body. With an ultrasound, the doctor can see the cyst's shape, size, location, and mass (if it is fluid-filled, solid, or mixed).

- **A Pregnancy Test:** This test may be given to rule out pregnancy.

- **Hormone Level Tests:** Hormone levels may be checked to see if there are hormone-related problems.

- **A Blood Test:** This test is done to find out if the cyst may be cancerous. The test measures a substance in the blood called cancer-antigen 125 (CA-125). The amount of CA-125 is higher with ovarian cancer. But some ovarian cancers don't make enough CA-125 to be detected by the test. Some noncancerous diseases also raise CA-125 levels. Those diseases include uterine fibroids and endometriosis. Noncancerous causes of higher CA-125 are more common in women younger than 35.

Ovarian cancer is very rare in this age group. The CA-125 test is most often given to women who are older than 35, at high risk for ovarian cancer, and have a cyst that is partly solid.

How are cysts treated?

Watchful Waiting: If you have a cyst, you may be told to wait and have a second exam in one to three months. Your doctor will check to see if the cyst has changed in size. This is a common treatment option for women who have these characteristics:

• Are in their childbearing years

• Have no symptoms

• Have a fluid-filled cyst

Surgery: Your doctor may want to remove the cyst if you are postmenopausal or if the cyst has these characteristics:

• Doesn't go away after several menstrual cycles

• Gets larger

• Looks odd on the ultrasound

• Causes pain

There are two main surgeries for ovarian cysts:

• **Laparoscopy:** Done if the cyst is small and looks benign (noncancerous) on the ultrasound. While you are under general anesthesia, a very small cut is made above or below your navel. A small instrument that acts like a telescope is put into your abdomen. Then your doctor can remove the cyst.

• **Laparotomy:** Done if the cyst is large and may be cancerous. While you are under general anesthesia, larger incisions are made in the stomach to remove the cyst. The cyst is then tested for cancer. If it is cancerous, the doctor may need to take out the ovary and other tissues, like the uterus. If only one ovary is taken out, your body is still fertile and can still produce estrogen.

Birth Control Pills: If you keep forming functional cysts, your doctor may prescribe birth control pills to stop you from ovulating. If you don't ovulate, you are less likely to form new cysts. You can also use Depo-Provera®. It is a hormone that is injected into muscle. It prevents ovulation for three months at a time.

Can ovarian cysts be prevented?

No, ovarian cysts cannot be prevented. The good news is that most cysts don't cause symptoms, are not cancerous, and go away on their own.

When are women most likely to have ovarian cysts?

Most functional ovarian cysts occur during childbearing years. And most of those cysts are not cancerous. Women who are past menopause (ages 50–70) with ovarian cysts have a higher risk of ovarian cancer. At any age, if you think you have a cyst, see your doctor for a pelvic exam.

✔ **Quick Tip**

Talk to your doctor or nurse if you notice:
changes in your period, pain in the pelvic area, or any of the
major symptoms of cysts.

Chapter 26

Endometriosis

What is endometriosis?

Endometriosis is a common health problem in women. It gets its name from the word endometrium, the tissue that lines the uterus or womb. Endometriosis occurs when this tissue grows outside of the uterus on other organs or structures in the body.

Most often, endometriosis is found on the ovaries, fallopian tubes, tissues that hold the uterus in place, outer surface of the uterus, and the lining of the pelvic cavity. Other sites for growths can include the vagina, cervix, vulva, bowel, bladder, or rectum. In rare cases, endometriosis has been found in other parts of the body, such as the lungs, brain, and skin.

What are the symptoms of endometriosis?

The most common symptom of endometriosis is pain in the lower abdomen or pelvis, or the lower back, mainly during menstrual periods. The amount of pain a woman feels does not depend on how much endometriosis she has. Some women have no pain, even though their disease affects large areas. Other women with endometriosis have severe pain even though they have only a few small growths.

About This Chapter: Information in this chapter is from "Endometriosis: Frequently Asked Questions," a publication of the U.S. Department of Health and Human Services, November 2009.

Symptoms of endometriosis can include the following:

• Very painful menstrual cramps; pain may get worse over time

• Chronic pain in the lower back and pelvis

• Pain during or after sex

• Intestinal pain

• Painful bowel movements or painful urination during menstrual periods

• Spotting or bleeding between menstrual periods

• Infertility or not being able to get pregnant

• Fatigue

• Diarrhea, constipation, bloating, or nausea, especially during menstrual periods

Recent research shows a link between other health problems in women with endometriosis and their families. The following are examples of some of these conditions:

• Allergies, asthma, and chemical sensitivities

• Autoimmune diseases, in which the body's system that fights illness attacks itself instead (such as hypothyroidism, multiple sclerosis, and lupus)

• Chronic fatigue syndrome (CFS) and fibromyalgia

• Being more likely to get infections and mononucleosis

• Mitral valve prolapse, a condition in which one of the heart's valves does not close as tightly as normal

• Frequent yeast infections

• Certain cancers, such as ovarian, breast, endocrine, kidney, thyroid, brain, and colon cancers, and melanoma and non-Hodgkin's lymphoma

Why does endometriosis cause pain and health problems?

Growths of endometriosis are benign (not cancerous). But they still can cause many problems. To see why, it helps to understand a woman's menstrual cycle. Every month, hormones cause the lining of a woman's uterus to build up with tissue and blood vessels. If a woman does not get pregnant, the uterus sheds this tissue and blood. It comes out of the body through the vagina as her menstrual period.

Patches of endometriosis also respond to the hormones produced during the menstrual cycle. With the passage of time, the growths of endometriosis may expand by adding extra tissue and blood. The symptoms of endometriosis often get worse.

Tissue and blood that is shed into the body can cause inflammation, scar tissue, and pain. As endometrial tissue grows, it can cover or grow into the ovaries and block the fallopian tubes. Trapped blood in the ovaries can form cysts, or closed sacs. It also can cause inflammation and cause the body to form scar tissue and adhesions, tissue that sometimes binds organs together. This scar tissue may cause pelvic pain and make it hard for women to get pregnant. The growths can also cause problems in the intestines and bladder.

What can raise my chances of getting endometriosis?

You might be more likely to get endometriosis if you have these characteristics:

- Never had children

- Menstrual periods that last more than seven days

- Short menstrual cycles (27 days or less)

- A family member (mother, aunt, sister) with endometriosis

- A health problem that prevents normal passage of menstrual blood flow

- Damage to cells in the pelvis from an infection

How can I reduce my chances of getting endometriosis?

There are no definite ways to lower your chances of getting endometriosis. Yet, since the hormone estrogen is involved in thickening the lining of the uterus during the menstrual cycle, you can try to lower levels of estrogen in your body.

✔ Quick Tip

To keep lower estrogen levels in your body, you can exercise regularly, keep a low amount of body fat, and avoid large amounts of alcohol and drinks with caffeine.

How do I know that I have endometriosis?

If you have symptoms of this disease, talk with your doctor or your obstetrician/gynecologist (OB/GYN). An OB/GYN has special training to diagnose and treat this condition. Sometimes endometriosis is mistaken for other health problems that cause pelvic pain and the exact cause might be hard to pinpoint.

The doctor will talk to you about your symptoms and health history. The doctor may also do these tests to check for clues of endometriosis:

Pelvic Exam: Your doctor will perform a pelvic exam to feel for large cysts or scars behind your uterus. Smaller areas of endometriosis are hard to feel.

Ultrasound: Your doctor could perform an ultrasound, an imaging test to see if there are ovarian cysts from endometriosis. During a vaginal ultrasound, the doctor will insert a wand-shaped scanner into your vagina. During an ultrasound of your pelvis, a scanner is moved across your abdomen. Both tests use sound waves to make pictures of your reproductive organs. Magnetic resonance imaging (MRI) is another common imaging test that can produce a picture of the inside of your body.

Laparoscopy: The only way for your doctor to know for sure that you have endometriosis is to look inside your abdomen to see endometriosis tissue. He or she can do this through a minor surgery called laparoscopy. You will receive general anesthesia before the surgery. Then, your abdomen is expanded with a gas to make it easy to see your organs. A tiny cut is made in your abdomen and a thin tube with a light is placed inside to see growths from endometriosis. Sometimes doctors can diagnose endometriosis just by seeing the growths. Other times, they need to take a small sample of tissue and study it under a microscope.

What causes endometriosis?

No one knows for sure what causes this disease, but experts have a number of theories:

- Since endometriosis runs in families, it may be carried in the genes, or some families have traits that make them more likely to get it.

- Endometrial tissue may move from the uterus to other body parts through the blood system or lymph system.

- If a woman has a faulty immune system it will fail to find and destroy endometrial tissue growing outside of the uterus. Recent research shows that immune system disorders and certain cancers are more common in women with endometriosis.

- The hormone estrogen appears to promote the growth of endometriosis. So, some research is looking at whether it is a disease of the endocrine system, the body's system of glands, hormones, and other secretions.

- Endometrial tissue has been found in abdominal scars and might have been moved there by mistake during a surgery.

- Small amounts of tissue from when a woman was an embryo might later become endometriosis.

✤ It's A Fact!!

If your doctor does not find signs of an ovarian cyst during an ultrasound, before doing a laparoscopy, your doctor may prescribe birth control pills to control your menstrual cycle. Sometimes this treatment helps lessen pelvic pain during your period.

Some doctors may offer another treatment that blocks the menstrual cycle and lowers the amount of estrogen your body makes before doing a laparoscopy. This treatment is a medicine called a gonadotropin releasing hormone (GnRH) agonist, which also may help pelvic pain. If your pain improves on this medicine, the doctor will likely think that you have endometriosis.

Laparoscopy is often recommended for diagnosis and treatment if the pelvic pain persists, even after taking birth control pills and pain medicine.

- New research shows a link between dioxin exposure and getting endometriosis. Dioxin is a toxic chemical from the making of pesticides and the burning of wastes. More research is needed to find out whether man-made chemicals cause endometriosis.

- Endometrial tissue may back up into the abdomen through the fallopian tubes during a woman's monthly period. This transplanted tissue could grow outside of the uterus. However, most experts agree that this theory does not entirely explain why endometriosis develops.

How is endometriosis treated?

There is no cure for endometriosis, but there are many treatments for the pain and infertility that it causes. Talk with your doctor about what option is best for you. The treatment you choose will depend on your symptoms, age, and plans for getting pregnant.

Pain Medication: For some women with mild symptoms, doctors may suggest taking over-the-counter medicines for pain. These include ibuprofen (Advil and Motrin) or naproxen (Aleve). When these medicines don't help, doctors may prescribe stronger pain relievers.

Hormone Treatment: When pain medicine is not enough, doctors often recommend hormone medicines to treat endometriosis. Only women who do not wish to become pregnant can use these drugs. Hormone treatment is best for women with small growths who do not have bad pain. Hormones come in many forms including pills, shots, and nasal sprays.

Surgery: Surgery is usually the best choice for women with severe endometriosis—many growths, a great deal of pain, or fertility problems. There are both minor and more complex surgeries that can help.

✔ Quick Tip

It is important to get support to cope with endometriosis. Consider joining a support group to talk with other women who have endometriosis. There are support groups on the internet and in many communities. It is also important to learn as much as you can about the disease. Talking with friends, family, and your doctor can help.

Chapter 27

Polycystic Ovary Syndrome (PCOS)

What is polycystic ovary syndrome (PCOS)?

PCOS is a health problem that can affect a woman's menstrual cycle, ability to have children, hormones, heart, blood vessels, and appearance.

With PCOS, women typically have these characteristics:

- High levels of androgens (sometimes called male hormones, though females also make them)
- Missed or irregular periods (monthly bleeding)
- Many small cysts (fluid-filled sacs) in their ovaries

How many women have PCOS?

Between one in 10 and one in 20 women of childbearing age has PCOS. As many as five million women in the United States may be affected. It can occur in girls as young as 11 years old.

What causes PCOS?

The cause of PCOS is unknown. But most experts think that several factors, including genetics, could play a role. Women with PCOS are more likely to have a mother or sister with PCOS.

About This Chapter: Information in this chapter is from "Polycystic Ovary Syndrome (PCOS): Frequently Asked Questions," a publication of the U.S. Department of Health and Human Services, March 2010.

A main underlying problem with PCOS is a hormonal imbalance. In women with PCOS, the ovaries make more androgens than normal. Androgens are male hormones that females also make. High levels of these hormones affect the development and release of eggs during ovulation.

What are the symptoms of PCOS?

The symptoms of PCOS can vary from woman to woman. These are some of the symptoms of PCOS:

• Infertility (not able to get pregnant) because of not ovulating

• Infrequent, absent, and/or irregular menstrual periods

• Hirsutism, or increased hair growth on the face, chest, stomach, back, thumbs, or toes

• Cysts on the ovaries

• Acne, oily skin, or dandruff

• Weight gain or obesity, usually with extra weight around the waist

• Male-pattern baldness or thinning hair

• Patches of skin on the neck, arms, breasts, or thighs that are thick and dark brown or black

• Skin tags—excess flaps of skin in the armpits or neck area

• Pelvic pain

• Anxiety or depression

• Sleep apnea, when breathing stops for short periods of time while asleep

---

✤ It's A Fact!!

Researchers also think insulin may be linked to PCOS. Insulin is a hormone that controls the change of sugar, starches, and other food into energy for the body to use or store. Many women with PCOS have too much insulin in their bodies because they have problems using it. Excess insulin appears to increase production of androgen. High androgen levels can lead to acne, excessive hair growth, weight gain, and problems with ovulation.

❖ It's A Fact!!
PCOS is the most common cause of female infertility.

Why do women with PCOS have trouble with their menstrual cycle and fertility?

The ovaries, where a woman's eggs are produced, have tiny fluid-filled sacs called follicles or cysts. As the egg grows, the follicle builds up fluid. When the egg matures, the follicle breaks open, the egg is released, and the egg travels through the fallopian tube to the uterus (womb) for fertilization. This is called ovulation. In women with PCOS, the ovary doesn't make all of the hormones it needs for an egg to fully mature. The follicles may start to grow and build up fluid but ovulation does not occur. Instead, some follicles may remain as cysts. For these reasons, ovulation does not occur and the hormone progesterone is not made. Without progesterone, a woman's menstrual cycle is irregular or absent. Plus, the ovaries make male hormones, which also prevent ovulation.

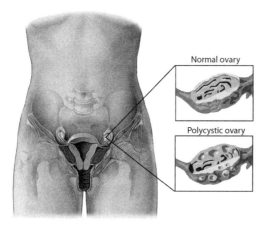

Figure 27.1. Normal Vs. Polycystic Ovaries.

How do I know if I have PCOS?

There is no single test to diagnose PCOS. Your doctor will take the following steps to find out if you have PCOS or if something else is causing your symptoms.

Medical History: Your doctor will ask about your menstrual periods, weight changes, and other symptoms.

Physical Exam: Your doctor will want to measure your blood pressure, body mass index (BMI), and waist size. He or she also will check the areas of increased hair growth. You should try to allow the natural hair to grow for a few days before the visit.

Pelvic Exam: Your doctor might want to check to see if your ovaries are enlarged or swollen by the increased number of small cysts.

Blood Tests: Your doctor may check the androgen hormone and glucose (sugar) levels in your blood.

Vaginal Ultrasound (Sonogram): Your doctor may perform a test that uses sound waves to take pictures of the pelvic area. It might be used to examine your ovaries for cysts and check the endometrium (lining of the womb). This lining may become thicker if your periods are not regular.

How is PCOS treated?

Because there is no cure for PCOS, it needs to be managed to prevent problems. Treatment goals are based on your symptoms, whether or not you want to become pregnant, and lowering your chances of getting heart disease and diabetes. Many women will need a combination of treatments to meet these goals. Some treatments for PCOS include:

Lifestyle Modification: Many women with PCOS are overweight or obese, which can cause health problems. You can help manage your PCOS by eating healthy and exercising to keep your weight at a healthy level.

Birth Control Pills: For women who don't want to get pregnant, birth control pills can control menstrual cycles, reduce male hormone levels, and help to clear acne.

✔ Quick Tip

Healthy eating tips include limiting processed foods and foods with added sugars and adding more whole-grain products, fruits, vegetables, and lean meats to your diet.

Diabetes Medications: The medicine metformin (Glucophage) is used to treat type 2 diabetes. It has also been found to help with PCOS symptoms, though it isn't approved by the U.S. Food and Drug Administration (FDA) for this use.

Fertility Medications: Lack of ovulation is usually the reason for fertility problems in women with PCOS. Several medications that stimulate ovulation can help women with PCOS become pregnant.

Surgery: Ovarian drilling is a surgery that may increase the chance of ovulation. It's sometimes used when a woman does not respond to fertility medicines.

Medicine For Increased Hair Growth Or Extra Male Hormones: Medicines called anti-androgens may reduce hair growth and clear acne. Spironolactone (Aldactone), first used to treat high blood pressure, has been shown to reduce the impact of male hormones on hair growth in women. Finasteride (Propecia), a medicine taken by men for hair loss, has the same effect. Anti-androgens are often combined with birth control pills. These medications should not be taken if you are trying to become pregnant.

Other Treatments: Some research has shown that bariatric (weight loss) surgery may be effective in resolving PCOS in morbidly obese women. Morbid obesity means having a BMI of more than 40, or a BMI of 35 to 40 with an obesity-related disease.

How does PCOS affect a woman while pregnant?

Women with PCOS appear to have higher rates of miscarriage, gestational diabetes, pregnancy-induced high blood pressure (preeclampsia), and premature delivery.

Babies born to women with PCOS have a higher risk of spending time in a neonatal intensive care unit or of dying before, during, or shortly after birth. Most of the time, these problems occur in multiple-birth babies (twins, triplets).

> ♣ **It's A Fact!!**
> Researchers are studying whether the diabetes medicine metformin can prevent or reduce the chances of having problems while pregnant.

Does PCOS put women at risk for other health problems?

Women with PCOS have greater chances of developing several serious health conditions, including life-threatening diseases. Recent studies found these relationships:

- More than 50 percent of women with PCOS will have diabetes or pre-diabetes (impaired glucose tolerance) before the age of 40.

- The risk of heart attack is four to seven times higher in women with PCOS than women of the same age without PCOS.

- Women with PCOS are at greater risk of having high blood pressure.

- Women with PCOS have high levels of LDL (bad) cholesterol and low levels of HDL (good) cholesterol.

- Women with PCOS may also develop anxiety and depression. It is important to talk to your doctor about treatment for these mental health conditions.

Women with PCOS are also at risk for endometrial cancer. Irregular menstrual periods and the lack of ovulation cause women to produce the hormone estrogen, but not the hormone progesterone. Progesterone causes the endometrium (lining of the womb) to shed each month as a menstrual period. Without progesterone, the endometrium becomes thick, which can cause heavy or irregular bleeding. Over time, this can lead to endometrial hyperplasia, when the lining grows too much, and cancer.

I have PCOS. What can I do to prevent complications?

If you have PCOS, get your symptoms under control at an earlier age to help reduce your chances of having complications like diabetes and heart disease. Talk to your doctor about treating all your symptoms, rather than focusing on just one aspect of your PCOS, such as problems getting pregnant. Also, talk to your doctor about getting tested for diabetes regularly.

How can I cope with the emotional effects of PCOS?

Having PCOS can be difficult. You may feel embarrassed by your appearance, worried about being able to get pregnant, or depressed. Getting treatment for PCOS can help with these concerns and help boost your self-esteem. You may also want to look for support groups in your area or online to help you deal with the emotional effects of PCOS. You are not alone and there are resources available for women with PCOS.

Chapter 28

Premature Ovarian Failure

What is premature ovarian failure?

The term premature ovarian failure describes a stop in the normal functioning of the ovaries in a woman younger than age 40. Some people also use the term primary ovarian insufficiency to describe this condition. It is also known as hypergonadotropic hypogonadism.

Health care providers used to call this condition premature menopause, but premature ovarian failure is actually much different than menopause. In menopause, a woman will likely never have another menstrual period again; women with premature ovarian failure are much more likely to get periods, even if they come irregularly. A woman in menopause has virtually no chance of getting pregnant; a woman with premature ovarian failure has a greatly reduced chance of getting pregnant, but pregnancy is still possible.

What are the symptoms of premature ovarian failure?

The most common first symptom of premature ovarian failure is skipping or having irregular periods. Some women with premature ovarian failure also have other symptoms, similar to those of women going through natural menopause. These may include symptoms such as the following:

About This Chapter: Information in this chapter is from "Premature Ovarian Failure," a publication of the National Institute of Child Health and Human Development, May 2007.

- Hot flashes and night sweats

- Irritability, poor concentration

- Decreased interest in sex or pain during sex

- Drying of the vagina

- Infertility

Premature ovarian failure also puts women at risk for some other health conditions, some of them serious:

- **Osteoporosis:** Loss of bone strength and bone density. Getting enough calcium, vitamin D, and weight-bearing physical activity can help reduce this risk.

- **Low Thyroid Function**: Affects metabolism and can cause very low energy. Replacing the thyroid hormone can treat the problem.

- **Addison Disease**: An autoimmune disorder in which the body has trouble handling physical stress, such an injury or illness, because of problems with the adrenal glands. About three percent of women with premature ovarian failure also have Addison disease. Addison disease can be dangerous for women who don't know they have it. This condition can't be prevented, but can be managed with help from your health care provider.

- **Heart Disease**: Estrogen replacement therapy, along with keeping a healthy body weight and getting regular moderate physical activity, can help reduce this risk.

✣ It's A Fact!!
It is important to know that people who are carriers for the gene for Fragile X syndrome, or who have the premutation for the condition, are more likely than other people to get premature ovarian failure. If you are a Fragile X carrier or have a premutation, it is important to get tested for premature ovarian failure.

Are there treatments for the symptoms of premature ovarian failure?

There is no proven treatment to make a woman's ovaries work normally again. However, there are treatments that can help some of the symptoms of premature ovarian failure.

- Estrogen replacement therapy (ERT), also called hormone replacement therapy (HRT) gives women the estrogen and other hormones their bodies are not making. HRT can help women have regular periods and lower their risk for osteoporosis.

- Current research is looking into giving women the hormone testosterone to help prevent bone loss in women with premature ovarian failure.

How is premature ovarian failure diagnosed?

Because one of the most common signs of premature ovarian failure is irregular periods, women should pay close attention to their menstrual cycles and tell their health care provider about any changes.

If your health care provider thinks you may have premature ovarian failure, he or she may do a blood test to measure the level of a hormone called follicle stimulating hormone that is normally present in the body. This test will help determine whether the ovaries are working properly or not.

What causes premature ovarian failure?

Researchers know that in women in premature ovarian failure something happens to stop the normal functioning of the ovaries but in most cases, the exact cause is not clear.

Most research focuses on a problem with the follicles in the ovaries. Follicles in the ovaries start out as microscopic seeds. These seeds mature into eggs, which travel to the uterus for fertilization. Follicles also release the hormone estrogen, which is important for a woman's overall health and bone health.

Most women have enough follicles to last until menopause. However, this may not be the case in women with premature ovarian failure. Women with premature ovarian failure may fall into one of two groups:

- A woman with follicle depletion has no follicles left in her ovaries and there is no way to make more.

- A woman with follicle dysfunction may have follicles in her ovaries, but they are not working properly.

About 10 percent to 20 percent of women with premature ovarian failure have a family history of the condition. This finding suggests that some cases of premature ovarian failure can be genetic. However, genetics is not the only cause of premature ovarian failure.

How does premature ovarian failure affect fertility?

Women with premature ovarian failure are unlikely to get pregnant because their ovaries do not work correctly. At this time there is no proven treatment to improve a woman's ability to have a baby naturally if she has premature ovarian failure.

However, between five percent and 10 percent of women with premature ovarian failure become pregnant without fertility treatment. There is also a type of fertility treatment known as egg donation which may be an option for women with premature ovarian failure.

Chapter 29

Lichen Sclerosus

What is lichen sclerosus?

Lichen sclerosus is a long-term problem of the skin. It mostly affects the genital and anal areas. Sometimes, lichen sclerosus appears on the upper body, breasts, and upper arms.

Who gets lichen sclerosus?

Lichen sclerosus appears in women, men, and children, but it is most common in women. It is uncommon in men and rare in children.

What are the symptoms?

Early in the disease, small white spots appear on the skin. The spots are usually shiny and smooth. Later, the spots grow into bigger patches. The skin on the patches becomes thin and crinkled. Then the skin tears easily, and bright red or purple bruises are common. Sometimes, the skin becomes scarred. If the disease is a mild case, there may be no symptoms.

There are sometimes other symptoms:

• Itching (very common)

• Discomfort or pain

About This Chapter: Information in this chapter is from "What Is Lichen Sclerosus?" a publication of the National Institute of Arthritis and Musculoskeletal and Skin Diseases, National Institutes of Health, June 2009.

- Bleeding

- Blisters

What causes lichen sclerosus?

Doctors don't know the exact cause of lichen sclerosus. Some doctors think an overactive immune system and hormone problems may play a role. It is also thought that people inherit the likelihood of getting the disease. Sometimes, lichen sclerosus appears on skin that has been damaged or scarred from some other previous injury.

> ✤ **It's A Fact!!**
> Lichen sclerosus is not contagious (it can't be caught from another person).

How is it diagnosed?

Doctors can look at severe lichen sclerosus and know what it is. But usually, a doctor takes a small piece of the skin patch (biopsy) and looks at it under a microscope. This allows doctors to make sure that it is not a different disease.

How is it treated?

If you have patches on the arms or upper body, they usually don't need treatment. The patches go away over time.

Lichen sclerosus of the genital skin should be treated. Even if it isn't painful or itchy, the patches can scar. This can cause problems with urination or sex. There is also a very small chance that skin cancer may develop in the patches.

Surgery is normally a good option for men. Circumcision (removing the foreskin on the penis) is the most widely used therapy for men with lichen sclerosus. The disease usually does not come back. Surgery is normally not a good option for women. When the lichen sclerosus patches are removed from the genitals of women and girls, they usually come back.

Treatment also includes using very strong cortisone cream or ointment on the skin. You put these creams on the patches every day for several weeks. This stops the itching. Then you use the cream or ointment two times a week for a long time to keep the disease from coming back. Treatment does not fix the scarring that may have already occurred. You need regular follow-up by a doctor because using these creams and ointments for a long time can cause side effects:

- Thinning and redness of the skin

- Stretch marks where the cream is applied

- Genital yeast infections

Sometimes, you don't get better when using the cortisone creams. Some things that can keep symptoms from clearing up are low estrogen levels, infection, and allergy to the medication.

When creams and ointments don't work, your doctor may suggest other treatments:

- Retinoids, or vitamin A-like drugs

- Tacrolimus ointment

- Ultraviolet light treatments (not used on skin of the genitals)

If a young girl gets lichen sclerosis, she may not require lifelong treatment. Lichen sclerosus sometimes goes away at puberty. Scarring and changes in skin color may remain.

Can people with lichen sclerosus have sex?

Women with severe lichen sclerosus in the genitals may not be able to have sex. The disease can cause scars that narrow the vagina. Also, sex can hurt and cause the patches to bleed. However, treatment with creams or ointments can help. Women with severe scarring in the vagina may need surgery, but only after lichen sclerosus is controlled with medication.

✔ Quick Tip

If you need medicine, ask your doctor these questions:
- How does the medicine work?
- What are its side effects?
- Why is it the best treatment for my lichen sclerosus?

Is lichen sclerosus related to cancer?

Lichen sclerosus does not cause skin cancer. However, skin that is scarred by lichen sclerosus is more likely to develop skin cancer. If you have the disease, see the doctor every six to 12 months. The doctor can look at and treat any changes in the skin.

What kind of doctor treats lichen sclerosus?

Lichen sclerosus is treated by one of the following types of physicians:

- Dermatologists (doctors who treat the skin)
- Gynecologists (doctors who treat the female reproductive system)
- Urologists (doctors who treat the urinary or urogenital tract)
- Primary health care providers

Chapter 30

Developmental Disorders Of The Vagina And Vulva

Developmental disorders of the vagina and vulva include many different structural problems that occur while the baby is developing in the mother's womb.

Causes

Abnormalities of the female vagina and vulva include:

Imperforate Hymen: The hymen is a thin tissue that partly covers the opening to the vagina. An imperforate hymen completely blocks the vaginal opening, so menstrual blood or mucus cannot flow out of the body. This often leads to painful swelling of the vagina. Sometimes the hymen has only a very small opening. This problem may not be discovered until puberty. Some baby girls are born without a hymen.

Vaginal Abnormalities: A baby girl may be born without a vagina or have the vaginal opening blocked by a layer of cells that are higher up in the vagina than where the hymen is. A missing vagina is most often due to Mayer-Rokitansky-Kuster-Hauser syndrome. In this syndrome, the baby is missing part or all of the internal reproductive organs (uterus, cervix, and fallopian tubes). Other abnormalities include having two vaginas or a vagina that opens into the urinary tract.

Problems With Outer (External) Genitals: Developmental problems may cause the folds of tissue around the opening of the vagina to join together. This is called a fused labia. Other developmental problems may lead to a swollen clitoris or ambiguous genitalia.

Symptoms

Symptoms may include:

- Inability to empty the bladder (urinary retention)
- Lack of menstrual periods
- Painful intercourse
- Pelvic pain that comes back

Exams And Tests

Finding problems with development early is important, especially when the gender is unclear (sexual ambiguity).

An examination of the outside (external) genitals may show:

- Enlarged clitoris
- One side of labia larger than the other, or unusually large on both sides
- Opening of the vagina very close to the urethra or anus
- Urethra located on the clitoris

An examination of the vagina may show:

- Abnormal "wall" of tissue (septum) in the vagina that may either partly or completely divide the vagina across or straight up and down
- Blockage of the opening of the vagina (imperforate hymen), and a bulge at the opening of the vagina
- Labia that is stuck together (fused labia)
- Missing or partially formed vagina

Treatment

- Counseling for the parents (and child, if necessary) to address concerns and provide guidance for the child's development

- Hormones (depending on the condition)

- Surgery when the child is a newborn or infant (or sometimes not until after puberty) to make the genitals match with the child's gender (with the expert advice of a geneticist or other specialist)

Outlook (Prognosis)

It helps to find the problem while the child is still a newborn. Getting all of these as soon as possible can provide the child with the best outcome:

- Chromosomal studies

- Expert advice

- Treatment of the physical, emotional, and social concerns

In the past, most hermaphrodites were raised as males because their outside (external) genitals looked more masculine. However, they can grow breasts, and many get their periods (menstruate). After removing the testicles with surgery, some hermaphrodites can become pregnant and deliver normal children.

Possible Complications

Complications can occur if the diagnosis is made late or is not correct.

It is possible for a child who has the outside (external) genitals of one gender to have internal sexual organs of the opposite sex. Sometimes, these internal sexual organs are at risk for cancer and must be surgically removed around the time of puberty.

When To Contact A Medical Professional

Call for an appointment with your health care provider if you notice:

- Abnormal genitals

- Menstruation does not begin at puberty

- Pubic hair or breasts do not develop at puberty

- Unexpected male traits

Prevention

There is no current way to prevent this condition.

✤ **It's A Fact!!**
Getting the right nutrition during pregnancy and avoiding exposure to illness, certain medications, and alcohol are all important for the baby to grow and develop. However, development problems may still occur, even if the mother makes every effort to ensure a healthy pregnancy.

Part Four

For Guys Only

Chapter 31

The Male Reproductive System

Ever wonder how the universe could allow the existence of someone as annoying as your bratty little brother or sister? The answer lies in reproduction. If people—like your parents (ew!)—didn't reproduce, families would die out and the human race would cease to exist.

All living things reproduce. Reproduction—the process by which organisms make more organisms like themselves—is one of the things that set living things apart from nonliving matter. But even though the reproductive system is essential to keeping a species alive, unlike other body systems it's not essential to keeping an individual alive.

In the human reproductive process, two kinds of sex cells, or gametes (pronounced: gah-meetz), are involved. The male gamete, or sperm, and the female gamete, the egg or ovum, meet in the female's reproductive system to create a new individual. Both the male and female reproductive systems are essential for reproduction.

Humans, like other organisms, pass certain characteristics of themselves to the next generation through their genes, the special carriers of human traits.

About This Chapter: Information in this chapter is from "Male Reproductive System," May 2010, reprinted with permission from www.kidshealth.org. Copyright © 2010 The Nemours Foundation. This information was provided by KidsHealth, one of the largest resources online for medically reviewed health information written for parents, kids, and teens. For more articles like this one, visit www.KidsHealth.org, or www.TeensHealth.org.

The genes parents pass along to their children are what make children similar to others in their family, but they are also what make each child unique. These genes come from the father's sperm and the mother's egg, which are produced by the male and female reproductive systems.

What Is The Male Reproductive System?

Most species have two sexes: male and female. Each sex has its own unique reproductive system. They are different in shape and structure, but both are specifically designed to produce, nourish, and transport either the egg or sperm.

Unlike the female, whose sex organs are located entirely within the pelvis, the male has reproductive organs, or genitals, that are both inside and outside the pelvis. The male genitals include:

• the testicles

• the duct system, which is made up of the epididymis and the vas deferens

• the accessory glands, which include the seminal vesicles and prostate gland

• the penis

In a guy who's reached sexual maturity, the two testicles (pronounced: tes-tih-kulz), or testes (pronounced: tes-teez), produce and store millions of tiny sperm cells. The testicles are oval-shaped and grow to be about two inches (five centimeters) in length and one inch (three centimeters) in diameter. The testicles are also part of the endocrine system because they produce hormones, including testosterone (pronounced: tes-tos-tuh-rone). Testosterone is a major part of puberty in guys, and as a guy makes his way through puberty, his testicles produce more and more of it.

✤ It's A Fact!!

Testosterone is the hormone that causes guys to develop deeper voices, bigger muscles, and body and facial hair, and it also stimulates the production of sperm.

Alongside the testicles are the epididymis (pronounced: ep-ih-did-uh-mus) and the vas deferens (pronounced: vas def-uh-runz), which make up the duct system of the male reproductive organs. The vas deferens is a muscular tube that passes upward alongside the testicles and transports the sperm-containing fluid called semen (pronounced: see-mun). The epididymis is a set of coiled tubes (one for each testicle) that connects to the vas deferens.

The epididymis and the testicles hang in a pouch-like structure outside the pelvis called the scrotum. This bag of skin helps to regulate the temperature of testicles, which need to be kept cooler than body temperature to produce sperm. The scrotum changes size to maintain the right temperature. When the body is cold, the scrotum shrinks and becomes tighter to hold in body heat. When it's warm, the scrotum becomes larger and more floppy to get rid of extra heat. This happens without a guy ever having to think about it. The

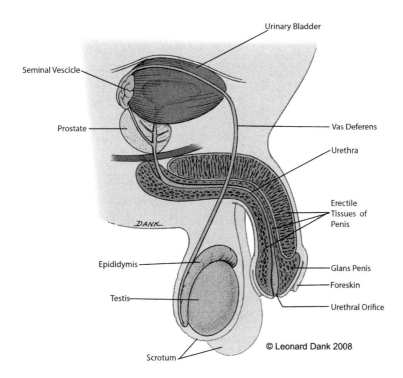

Figure 31.1. Male Reproductive System.

brain and the nervous system give the scrotum the cue to change size.

The accessory glands, including the seminal vesicles and the prostate gland, provide fluids that lubricate the duct system and nourish the sperm. The seminal vesicles are sac-like structures attached to the vas deferens to the side of the bladder. The prostate gland, which produces some of the parts of semen, surrounds the ejaculatory ducts at the base of the urethra (pronounced: yoo-ree-thruh), just below the bladder. The urethra is the channel that carries the semen to the outside of the body through the penis. The urethra is also part of the urinary system because it is also the channel through which urine passes as it leaves the bladder and exits the body.

> ♣ **It's A Fact!!**
> Boys who have circumcised penises and those who don't are no different: All penises work and feel the same, regardless of whether the foreskin has been removed.

The penis is actually made up of two parts: the shaft and the glans. The shaft is the main part of the penis and the glans is the tip (sometimes called the head). At the end of the glans is a small slit or opening, which is where semen and urine exit the body through the urethra. The inside of the penis is made of a spongy tissue that can expand and contract.

All boys are born with a foreskin, a fold of skin at the end of the penis covering the glans. Some boys have a circumcision, which means that a doctor or clergy member cuts away the foreskin. Circumcision is usually performed during a baby boy's first few days of life. Although circumcision is not medically necessary, parents who choose to have their children circumcised often do so based on religious beliefs, concerns about hygiene, or cultural or social reasons.

What Does The Male Reproductive System Do?

The male sex organs work together to produce and release semen into the reproductive system of the female during sexual intercourse. The male reproductive system also produces sex hormones, which help a boy develop into a sexually mature man during puberty.

When a baby boy is born, he has all the parts of his reproductive system in place, but it isn't until puberty that he is able to reproduce. When puberty begins, usually between the ages of 10 and 14, the pituitary (pronounced: pih-too-uh-ter-ee) gland—which is located near the brain—secretes hormones that stimulate the testicles to produce testosterone. The production of testosterone brings about many physical changes.

Although the timing of these changes is different for every guy, the stages of puberty generally follow a set sequence:

- During the first stage of male puberty, the scrotum and testes grow larger.

- Next, the penis becomes longer, and the seminal vesicles and prostate gland grow.

- Hair begins to appear in the pubic area and later it grows on the face and underarms. During this time, a male's voice also deepens.

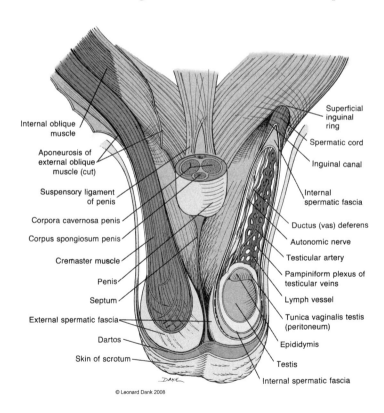

© Leonard Dank 2008

Figure 31.2. Spermatic Cord.

- Boys also undergo a growth spurt during puberty as they reach their adult height and weight.

Once a guy has reached puberty, he will produce millions of sperm cells every day. Each sperm is extremely small: only 1/600 of an inch (0.05 millimeters long). Sperm develop in the testicles within a system of tiny tubes called the seminiferous tubules (pronounced: sem-uh-nih-fuh-rus too-byoolz). At birth, these tubules contain simple round cells, but during puberty, testosterone and other hormones cause these cells to transform into sperm cells. The cells divide and change until they have a head and short tail, like tadpoles. The head contains genetic material (genes). The sperm use their tails to push themselves into the epididymis, where they complete their development.

The sperm then move to the vas deferens, or sperm duct. The seminal vesicles and prostate gland produce a whitish fluid called seminal fluid, which mixes with sperm to form semen when a male is sexually stimulated. The penis, which usually hangs limp, becomes hard when a male is sexually excited. Tissues in the penis fill with blood and it becomes stiff and erect (an erection). The rigidity of the erect penis makes it easier to insert into the female's vagina during sexual intercourse. When the erect penis is stimulated, muscles around the reproductive organs contract and force the semen through the duct system and urethra. Semen is pushed out of the male's body through his urethra—this process is called ejaculation. Each time a guy ejaculates, it can contain up to 500 million sperm.

> ♣ **It's A Fact!!**
> It takes sperm about four to six weeks to travel through the epididymis.

When the male ejaculates during intercourse, semen is deposited into the female's vagina. From the vagina the sperm make their way up through the cervix and move through the uterus with help from uterine contractions. If a mature egg is in one of the female's fallopian tubes, a single sperm may penetrate it, and fertilization, or conception, occurs.

This fertilized egg is now called a zygote (pronounced: zy-goat) and contains 46 chromosomes—half from the egg and half from the sperm. The genetic material from the male and female has combined so that a new individual can be created. The zygote divides again and again as it grows in the female's uterus, maturing over the course of the pregnancy into an embryo, a fetus, and finally a newborn baby.

Problems Affecting The Male Reproductive System

Guys may sometimes experience reproductive system problems. Below are some examples of disorders that affect the male reproductive system:

Disorders Of The Scrotum, Testicles, Or Epididymis

Conditions affecting the scrotal contents may involve the testicles, epididymis, or the scrotum itself.

- **Testicular Injury:** Even a mild injury to the testicles can cause severe pain, bruising, or swelling. Most testicular injuries occur when the testicles are struck, hit, kicked, or crushed, usually during sports or due to other trauma. Testicular torsion (pronounced: tor-zhun), when one of the testicles twists around, cutting off its blood supply, is also a problem that some teen guys experience—although it's not common.

- **Varicocele (Pronounced: Var-uh-koh-seal):** This is a varicose vein (an abnormally swollen vein) in the network of veins that run from the testicles. Varicoceles commonly develop while a guy is going through puberty. A varicocele is usually not harmful, although in some people it may damage the testicle or decrease sperm production, so it helps for a guy to see his doctor if he's concerned about changes in his testicles.

- **Testicular Cancer:** This is one of the most common cancers in men younger than 40. It occurs when cells in the testicle divide abnormally and form a tumor. Testicular cancer can spread to other parts of the body, but if it's detected early, the cure rate is excellent. All guys should perform testicular self-examinations regularly to help with early detection.

- **Epididymitis (Pronounced: Ep-uh-did-ih-my-tus)** is inflammation of the epididymis, the coiled tubes that connect the testes with the

---

✔ Quick Tip

If you think you have symptoms of a problem with your reproductive system or if you have questions about your growth and development, talk to your parent or doctor—many problems with the male reproductive system can be treated.

---

vas deferens. It is usually caused by an infection, such as the sexually transmitted disease chlamydia, and results in pain and swelling next to one of the testicles.

• **Hydrocele:** A hydrocele (pronounced: high-druh-seel) occurs when fluid collects in the membranes surrounding the testes. Hydroceles may cause swelling in the scrotum around the testicle but are generally painless. In some cases, surgery may be needed to correct the condition.

• **Inguinal Hernia:** When a portion of the intestines pushes through an abnormal opening or weakening of the abdominal wall and into the groin or scrotum, it is known as an inguinal (pronounced: in-gwuh-nul) hernia. The hernia may look like a bulge or swelling in the groin area. It can be corrected with surgery.

Disorders Of The Penis

Disorders affecting the penis include the following:

• **Inflammation Of The Penis:** Symptoms of penile inflammation include redness, itching, swelling, and pain. Balanitis occurs when the glans (the head of the penis) becomes inflamed. Posthitis is foreskin inflammation, which is usually due to a yeast or bacterial infection.

• **Hypospadias** is a disorder in which the urethra opens on the underside of the penis, not at the tip.

Chapter 32

Circumcision

What Is Circumcision?

At birth, baby boys have loose skin that covers the head of the penis. This is called the "foreskin." When all or part of the foreskin of the penis is cut off, it is called "circumcision."

Why Is Circumcision Done?

Circumcision is done for religious, cultural, appearance, or health reasons. Some religious groups circumcise boys. Persons who are Jewish believe that circumcision of baby boys at eight days old is a commandment from God and therefore, circumcision is a faith-based practice. Muslim people also believe that circumcision of boys is a way to be more faithful to God. In the Muslim faith, circumcision can be done at any point in a boy's life, depending on local traditions. Some parents choose circumcision so that their son will have a penis that looks like his father's. Other people choose circumcision because they believe it is cleaner or will protect the boy or man from infection or cancer.

About This Chapter: Information in this chapter is reprinted with permission from the *Journal of Midwifery and Women's Health*, Volume 52, Number 5, September/October 2007. Jennifer Shark and Amber Knoche, "Circumcision," 517–518. Copyright 2007 American College of Nurse-Midwives.

Is Circumcision Cleaner? Does It Protect From Infection Or Cancer?

Regular washing with soap and water will keep any penis clean. Circumcision does not make the penis cleaner. Uncircumcised boys do need to be taught to clean beneath their foreskin, just like they need to be taught to wash their hands or brush their teeth.

Circumcision does seem to protect against some types of infection or cancer. Cancer of the penis is one type of cancer that circumcision may prevent. However, cancer of the penis is very rare. Three hundred thousand circumcisions would need to be done to prevent one case. See the end of this chapter for more information on the risks and benefits of circumcision.

What Happens During A Circumcision?

Your health care provider will typically perform the circumcision in the hospital before you go home. Religious circumcisions are most often done at home or in a synagogue. Before the procedure, some providers inject a small amount of anesthesia at the base of the penis to block the pain. If you have a Jewish religious circumcision, your baby may be given a few drops of sweetened wine in a nipple just before the procedure.

✤ It's A Fact!!
Penis Care (Uncircumcised)

An uncircumcised penis is one with its foreskin intact. An infant boy with an uncircumcised penis requires no special care. Normal bathing is enough to keep it clean.

It is NOT recommended to pull back (retract) the foreskin for cleaning during infancy and childhood. This may injure the foreskin and cause scarring that could make retraction painful and difficult later in life.

Teenage boys should be taught to gently retract the foreskin during bathing and clean the penis thoroughly. After cleaning the penis, dry the area completely. Then, it is very important to pull the foreskin back over the head of the penis. Otherwise, the foreskin can slightly constrict the head of the penis, causing swelling and pain, called paraphimosis. This requires medical treatment.

Source: "Penis care (uncircumcised)," © 2010 A.D.A.M., Inc. Reprinted with permission.

There are different ways to do a circumcision. In one type, a clamp placed around the head of the penis cuts off the blood supply to the foreskin and the foreskin above the clamp is cut off. The clamp is left on the penis until the area heals and it falls off a few days later. In another type of circumcision, the foreskin is cut off with scissors or a scalpel.

After the circumcision, petroleum jelly and sometimes gauze may be put over the wound. This protects the end of the penis while it heals.

Who Chooses Circumcision?

Many people in the United States choose to circumcise their boys because they believe that a circumcised penis is cleaner than an uncircumcised one, which is not necessarily true: soap and water will keep any penis clean.

What Are The Risks And Benefits Of Circumcision?

People have strong feelings about circumcision. We do not have a lot of good information about the risks and benefits.

Possible Risks

- About one in 500 baby boys will have a problem with circumcision. Problems include:
    - bleeding or infection in the penis
    - infection spreading to other parts of the body
    - narrowing of the opening of the penis, which can cause problems with urination
    - partial amputation of the penis
    - death of some of the other skin on the penis
    - removal of too much foreskin, which can cause pain during sex later in life
    - very rarely, death. This occurs in about one in 500,000 boys
- We do not know much about pain in newborn babies. People used to think babies did not really feel pain. Now we know that they do. Many baby boys appear to feel a lot of pain during circumcision if anesthesia is not used.

• When older boys or men are circumcised, they have the same risks as babies. They report severe pain.

Possible Benefits

• Less risk for some kinds of cancers, like cancer of the penis

• Fewer bladder or kidney infections

• Less risk for some sexually transmitted infections, like human immunodeficiency virus (HIV)

For More Information

The American Academy of Family Physicians has great information about circumcision: www.familydoctor.org/042.xml

Medline plus has more detailed information about circumcision: www.nlm.nih.gov/medlineplus/circumcision.html

The American Academy of Pediatrics policy statement on circumcision: http://aappolicy.aappublications.org/cgi/content/full/pediatrics%3b103/3/686

Chapter 33

Penis Development

Is my penis normal?

Just about every guy wonders how he measures up in the "down-there" department at one time or another. Here's the lowdown for any guy who's ever worried about whether his penis is a normal size.

There's a fairly wide range of normal penis sizes—just as there is for every other body part. And just like other parts of the body, how a penis appears at different stages of a guy's life varies quite a bit. You wouldn't expect someone who is 11 years old to look the same as someone who's 19.

Guys normally develop at different times. Some may start developing as early as nine. Others may not start developing until 15 or even later. The age at which a guy starts to grow varies from person to person. It all depends on when he enters puberty and his hormones start doing their thing.

Growth in penis size is just one part of puberty, which also includes such changes as pubic hair development, testicular growth, muscle development, and a growth spurt. Late starters almost always catch up fine—they just reach full maturity a little later.

Penises come in different sizes, shapes, and colors. These traits are heredi-tary, like eye color or foot size, and there's nothing you can do to change them. Despite what you may hear or read, no special exercises, supplements, or diets will speed up the development process or change a guy's size. Also, like his feet, a guy's penis may appear smaller to him just because the perspective is different when he's looking down. And there's a lot less difference in penis size between guys when they get an erection than when their penises are relaxed.

In addition to size, guys also wonder about other aspects of how their penises look, such as whether the skin covering the penis is normal or if it's OK for a guy's penis to hang to the left or right (it is!). If you're concerned about how your penis looks, ask your doctor. Guys who are reaching puberty should have regular testicular exams, so that's a good time to ask your doctor any questions.

❖ It's A Fact!!

Chances are that you had a "wet dream"—something that can be embarrass-ing and confusing to teen guys, but is completely normal. A wet dream is also known as a nocturnal emission. Nocturnal means "at night" and emission means "discharge." This makes sense because a wet dream is when semen (the fluid con-taining sperm) is discharged from the penis during ejaculation while a guy's asleep. Usually wet dreams occur during dreams that have sexual images. Sometimes guys wake up from a wet dream, but sometimes they sleep through it.

Wet dreams begin during puberty when the body starts making more tes-tosterone, the major male hormone. Although some guys may feel embarrassed or even guilty about having wet dreams, they can't be controlled and you can't stop them from happening—most guys experience them at some point during puberty and even sometimes as adults.

Source: "What Are Wet Dreams?," May 2009, reprinted with permission from www.kid-shealth.org. Copyright © 2009 The Nemours Foundation. This information was provided by KidsHealth, one of the largest resources online for medically reviewed health information written for parents, kids, and teens. For more articles like this one, visit www.KidsHealth.org, or www.TeensHealth.org.

Taking a ride on the hormonal roller-coaster means lots of changes—and a lot of common worries—for both guys and girls. Just as guys may wonder about how their penises develop, lots of girls ask the same thing about their breasts.

If you're wondering about your development, don't try to compare yourself to your older brother or your best friend—they're probably at a different stage of development than you are anyway. The important thing to remember is that it's OK to not be a mirror image of the guy at the next urinal.

Chapter 34

Priapism

Priapism is a persistent, usually painful, erection that lasts for more than four hours and occurs without sexual stimulation. The condition develops when blood in the penis becomes trapped and is unable to drain. If the condition is not treated immediately, it can lead to scarring and permanent erectile dysfunction.

Priapism can occur in all age groups, including newborns. However, it usually affects men between the ages of 5 to 10 years and 20 to 50 years.

There are two categories of priapism: low-flow and high-flow.

- **Low-Flow:** This type of priapism is the result of blood being trapped in the erection chambers. It often occurs without a known cause in men who are otherwise healthy, but also affects men with sickle cell disease, leukemia (cancer of the blood), or malaria.

- **High-Flow:** High-flow priapism is more rare than low-flow and is usually not painful. It is the result of a ruptured artery from an injury to the penis or the perineum (area between the scrotum and anus), which prevents blood in the penis from circulating normally.

About This Chapter: Information in this chapter is from "Priapism," © 2010 The Cleveland Clinic Foundation, 9500 Euclid Avenue, Cleveland, OH 44195. All rights reserved. Reprinted with permission. Additional information is available from the Cleveland Clinic Health Information Center, 216-444-3771, toll-free 800-223-2273 extension 43771, or at http://my.clevelandclinic.org/health.

What causes priapism?

- **Sickle Cell Anemia:** Some adult cases of priapism are the result of sickle cell disease; approximately 42% of all adults with sickle cell will eventually develop priapism.

- **Medications:** A common cause of priapism is the use and/or misuse of medications. Drug-related priapism includes drugs such as Desyrel (used to treat depression) or Thorazine (used to treat certain mental illnesses). For people who have erectile dysfunction, injection therapy medications to treat the condition may also cause priapism.

Other causes of priapism include:

- trauma to the spinal cord or to the genital area
- black widow spider bites
- carbon monoxide poisoning
- illicit drug use, such as marijuana and cocaine

How is priapism diagnosed?

If you experience priapism, it is important that you seek medical care immediately. Tell your doctor:

- the length of time you have had the erection
- how long your erection usually lasts
- any medication or drugs, legal or illegal, that you have used. Be honest with your doctor; illegal drug use is particularly relevant since both marijuana and cocaine have been linked to priapism.
- whether or not priapism followed trauma to that area of the body

Your doctor will review your medical history and perform a physical examination to help determine the cause of priapism.

After the physical exam is complete, the doctor will take a blood-gas measurement of the blood from the penis. During this test, a small needle is placed in the penis, some of the blood is drawn, and then it is sent to a lab for analysis. This provides a clue as to the type of priapism, how long the condition has been present, and how much damage has occurred.

How is priapism treated?

The goal of all treatment is to make the erection go away and preserve future erectile function. If a person receives treatment within four to six hours, the erection can almost always be reduced with medication. If the erection has lasted less than four hours, decongestant medications, which may act to decrease blood flow to the penis, may be very helpful. Other treatment options include:

- **Ice Packs:** Ice applied to the penis and perineum may reduce swelling.

- **Surgical Ligation:** Used in some cases where an artery has been ruptured. The doctor will ligate (tie off) the artery that is causing the priapism in order to restore normal blood flow.

- **Intracavernous Injection:** Used for low-flow priapism. During this treatment, drugs known as alpha-agonists are injected into the penis. These drugs cause the veins to narrow, reducing blood flow to the penis and causing the swelling to subside.

- **Surgical Shunt:** Also used for low-flow priapism, a shunt is a passage-way that is surgically inserted into the penis to divert the blood flow and allow circulation to return to normal.

- **Aspiration:** After numbing the penis, doctors will insert a needle and drain blood from the penis to reduce pressure and swelling.

What is the outlook for people with priapism?

As long as treatment is prompt, the outlook for most people is very good. However, the longer medical attention is delayed, the greater the risk of permanent erectile dysfunction.

Chapter 35

Peyronie Disease

What is Peyronie disease?

Peyronie disease is characterized by a plaque, or hard lump, that forms within the penis. The plaque, a flat plate of scar tissue, develops on the top or bottom side of the penis inside a thick membrane called the tunica albuginea, which envelopes the erectile tissues. The plaque begins as a localized inflammation and develops into a hardened scar. This plaque has no relationship to the plaque that can develop in arteries.

Cases of Peyronie disease range from mild to severe. Symptoms may develop slowly or appear overnight. In severe cases, the hardened plaque reduces flexibility, causing pain and forcing the penis to bend or arc during erection. In many cases, the pain decreases over time, but the bend in the penis may remain a problem, making sexual intercourse difficult. The sexual problems that result can disrupt a couple's physical and emotional relationship and can lower a man's self-esteem. In a small percentage of men with the milder form of the disease, inflammation may resolve without causing significant pain or permanent bending.

About This Chapter: Information in this chapter is from "Peyronie's Disease," a publication of the National Institute of Diabetes and Digestive and Kidney Diseases (NIDDK). The NIDDK is part of the National Institutes of Health of the U.S. Department of Health and Human Services. NIH Publication No. 09–3902. April 2009.

A plaque on the topside of the shaft, which is most common, causes the penis to bend upward; a plaque on the underside causes it to bend downward. In some cases, the plaque develops on both top and bottom, leading to indentation and shortening of the penis. At times, pain, bending, and emotional distress prohibit sexual intercourse.

✤ **It's A Fact!!**
The plaque itself is benign, or noncancerous. It is not a tumor. Peyronie disease is not contagious and is not known to be caused by any transmittable disease.

Estimates of the prevalence of Peyronie disease range from less than one percent to 23 percent. A recent study in Germany found Peyronie disease in 3.2 percent of men between 30 and 80 years of age. Although the disease occurs mostly in middle age, younger and older men can develop it. About 30 percent of men with Peyronie disease develop hardened tissue on other parts of the body, such as the hand or foot. A common example is a condition known as Dupuytren's contracture of the hand. In some cases, Peyronie disease runs in families, which suggests that genetic factors might make a man vulnerable to the disease.

How does Peyronie disease develop?

Many researchers believe the plaque of Peyronie disease develops following trauma, such as hitting or bending, that causes localized bleeding inside the penis. Two chambers known as the corpora cavernosa run the length of the penis. A connecting tissue, called a septum, runs between the two chambers and attaches at the top and bottom of the tunica albuginea.

✤ **It's A Fact!!**

A French surgeon, François de la Peyronie, first described Peyronie disease in 1743. The problem was noted in print as early as 1687. Early writers classified it as a form of impotence, now called erectile dysfunction (ED). Peyronie disease can be associated with ED—the inability to achieve or sustain an erection firm enough for intercourse. However, experts now recognize ED as only one factor associated with the disease—a factor that is not always present.

If the penis is bumped or bent, an area where the septum attaches to the tunica albuginea may stretch beyond a limit, injuring the tunica albuginea and rupturing small blood vessels. As a result of aging, diminished elasticity near the point of attachment of the septum might increase the chances of injury. In addition, the septum can also be damaged and form tough, fibrous tissue, called fibrosis.

The tunica albuginea has many layers, and little blood flows through those layers. Therefore, the inflammation can be trapped between the layers for many months. During that time, the inflammatory cells may release substances that cause excessive fibrosis and reduce elasticity. This chronic process eventually forms a plaque with excessive amounts of scar tissue and causes calcification, loss of elasticity in spots, and penile deformity.

❖ **It's A Fact!!**
Some researchers theorize that Peyronie disease may be an auto-immune disorder.

While trauma might explain some cases of Peyronie disease, it does not explain why most cases develop slowly and with no apparent traumatic event. It also does not explain why some cases resolve or why similar conditions such as Dupuytren's contracture do not seem to result from severe trauma.

How is Peyronie disease evaluated?

Doctors can usually diagnose Peyronie disease based on a physical examination. The plaque can be felt when the penis is limp. Full evaluation, however, may require examination during erection to determine the severity of the deformity. The erection may be induced by injecting medicine into the penis or through self-stimulation. Some patients may eliminate the need to induce an erection in the doctor's office by taking a digital or Polaroid picture at home. The examination may include an ultrasound scan of the penis to pinpoint the location(s) and calcification of the plaque. The ultrasound can also be used to evaluate blood flow into and out of the penis if there is a concern about erectile dysfunction.

How is Peyronie disease treated?

Men with Peyronie disease usually seek medical attention because of painful erections, penile deformity, or difficulty with intercourse. Because the cause of

Peyronie disease and its development are not well understood, doctors treat the disease empirically; that is, they prescribe and continue methods that seem to help. The goal of therapy is to restore and maintain the ability to have intercourse. Providing education about the disease and its course often is all that is required. No strong evidence shows that any treatment other than surgery is universally effective. Experts usually recommend surgery only in long-term cases in which the disease is stabilized and the deformity prevents intercourse.

Because the course of Peyronie disease is different in each patient and because some patients experience improvement without treatment, medical experts suggest waiting one year or longer before having surgery. During that wait, patients often are willing to undergo treatments whose effectiveness has not been proven.

Medical Treatments: Researchers conducted small-scale studies in which men with Peyronie disease who were given vitamin E orally reported improvements. Yet, no controlled studies have established the effectiveness of vitamin E therapy. Similar inconclusive success has been attributed to aminobenzoate potassium (Potaba). Other oral medications that have been used include colchicine, tamoxifen, and pentoxifylline. Again, no controlled studies have been conducted on these medications.

Researchers have also tried injecting chemical agents such as verapamil, collagenase, steroids, and interferon alpha-2b directly into the plaques. Verapamil and interferon alpha-2b seem to diminish curvature of the penis. The other injectable agent, collagenase, is undergoing clinical trial and results are not yet available. Steroids, such as cortisone, have produced unwanted side effects, such as the atrophy or death of healthy tissues. Another intervention involves iontophoresis, the use of a painless current of electricity to deliver verapamil or some other agent under the skin into the plaque.

Radiation therapy, in which high-energy rays are aimed at the plaque, has also been used. Like some of the chemical treatments, radiation appears to reduce pain, but it has no effect on the plaque itself and can cause unwelcome side effects such as erectile dysfunction. Although the variety of agents and methods used points to the lack of a proven treatment, new insights into the wound healing process may one day yield more effective therapies.

Surgery: Three surgical procedures for Peyronie disease have had some success. One procedure involves removing or cutting of the plaque and attaching a patch of skin, vein, or material made from animal organs. This method may straighten the penis and restore some lost length from Peyronie disease. However, some patients may experience numbness of the penis and loss of erectile function.

A second procedure, called plication, involves removing or pinching a piece of the tunica albuginea from the side of the penis opposite the plaque, which cancels out the bending effect. This method is less likely to cause numbness or erectile dysfunction, but it cannot restore length or girth of the penis.

A third surgical option is to implant a device that increases rigidity of the penis. In some cases, an implant alone will straighten the penis adequately. If the implant alone does not straighten the penis, implantation is combined with one of the other two surgical procedures.

Most types of surgery produce positive results. But because complications can occur, and because many of the effects of Peyronie disease—for example, shortening of the penis—are not usually corrected by surgery, most doctors prefer to perform surgery only on the small number of men with curvature severe enough to prevent sexual intercourse.

♣ It's A Fact!!
Hope Through Research

Researchers from universities and government agencies are working to understand the causes of Peyronie disease. The National Institute of Diabetes and Digestive and Kidney Diseases (NIDDK) supports a project designed to define a common process that causes fibrosis in the penis and arterial stiffness—or arteriosclerosis—throughout the body. By studying this process at a cellular and molecular level, researchers hope to develop an effective therapy.

Chapter 36

Balanitis, Phimosis, And Paraphimosis

Balanitis

Balanitis is an inflammation of the foreskin and head of the penis.

Causes

Balanitis is usually caused by poor hygiene in uncircumcised men. The inflammation can be due to infection, harsh soaps, or failure to properly rinse soap off while bathing. Several other diseases, including reactive arthritis and lichen sclerosis et atrophicus, can lead to balanitis. Men with uncontrolled diabetes are at risk of developing balanitis.

Symptoms

- Redness of foreskin or penis

- Other rashes on the head of the penis

- Foul-smelling discharge

- Painful penis and foreskin

Exams And Tests

Your dermatologist or urologist may be able to diagnosis the cause of your balanitis by examination alone. However, additional skin tests for viruses, fungi, or bacteria are often needed. Occasionally, a skin biopsy is required.

Treatment

Treatment depends on the cause of the balanitis. For example, infectious balanitis may be treated with antibiotic pills or creams. Balanitis occurring with skin diseases may respond to steroid creams.

Outlook (Prognosis)

Most cases of balanitis can be controlled with medicated creams and good hygiene. Surgery is not usually necessary. Outcomes are nearly always positive.

> ♣ **It's A Fact!!**
> In severe cases, circumcision may be the best option.

Possible Complications

Chronic inflammation or infection can:

• scar and narrow the opening of the penis (meatal stricture)

• make it difficult and painful to retract the foreskin to expose the tip of the penis (a condition called phimosis)

• make it difficult to reposition the foreskin over the head of the penis (a condition called paraphimosis); swelling can affect the blood supply to the tip of the penis

When To Contact A Medical Professional

Notify your health care provider if you are experiencing any signs of balanitis including swelling of the foreskin or pain.

Prevention

Good hygiene can prevent most cases of balanitis. During bathing, the foreskin should be retracted to adequately clean and dry the area beneath it.

Phimosis And Paraphimosis

Phimosis

In phimosis, the foreskin is tight and cannot be retracted over the glans penis (the cone-shaped end of the penis). This condition is normal in newborns and young boys and usually resolves without treatment by about age five. In older men, phimosis may result from prolonged irritation or recurring balanoposthitis. The tightened foreskin can interfere with urination and sexual activity and may increase the risk of urinary tract infections. The usual treatment is circumcision. However, in children, sometimes the application of a corticosteroid cream two or three times daily and periodic gentle stretching of the foreskin are effective and spare the child a circumcision. The cream may be used for up to three months.

Paraphimosis

In paraphimosis, the retracted foreskin cannot be pulled forward to cover the glans penis. The condition most commonly develops when the foreskin is left retracted after a medical procedure (such as catheterization) or after cleaning the penis of a child. The glans penis swells, increasing pressure on the retracted foreskin, which then becomes trapped. The increasing pressure eventually prevents blood from reaching the penis, which could result in the destruction of penile tissue if the foreskin is not pulled back forward. Immediate treatment involves squeezing the glans penis to shrink it so that the foreskin can be pulled forward. If this technique does not work, the penis is anesthetized and the foreskin is slit to relieve the constriction. Later, circumcision is done.

Chapter 37

Penile Cancer

General Information About Penile Cancer

Penile cancer is a disease in which malignant (cancer) cells form in the tissues of the penis. The penis is a rod-shaped male reproductive organ that passes sperm and urine from the body. It contains two types of erectile tissue (spongy tissue with blood vessels that fill with blood to make an erection):

- **Corpora Cavernosa:** The two columns of erectile tissue that form most of the penis.

- **Corpus Spongiosum:** The single column of erectile tissue that forms a small portion of the penis. The corpus spongiosum surrounds the urethra (the tube through which urine and sperm pass from the body).

Risk Factors

Anything that increases your chance of getting a disease is called a risk factor. Having a risk factor does not mean that you will get cancer; not having risk factors doesn't mean that you will not get cancer. People who think they may be at risk should discuss this with their doctor. Risk factors for penile cancer include the following:

About This Chapter: Information in this chapter is from "Penile Cancer Treatment (PDQ®)—Patient Version." PDQ® Cancer Information Summary. National Cancer Institute; Bethesda, MD. Updated 01/2010. Available at: http://www.cancer.gov. Accessed October 2010.

- Being age 60 or older

- Having phimosis (a condition in which the foreskin of the penis cannot be pulled back over the glans)

- Having poor personal hygiene

- Having many sexual partners

- Using tobacco products

> ❖ **It's A Fact!!**
> The erectile tissue is wrapped in connective tissue and covered with skin. The glans (head of the penis) is covered with loose skin called the foreskin.

Symptoms

Possible signs of penile cancer include sores, discharge, and bleeding. These and other symptoms may be caused by penile cancer. Other conditions may cause the same symptoms. A doctor should be consulted if you experience redness, irritation, or a sore or lump on the penis.

Diagnosis

Tests that examine the penis are used to detect (find) and diagnose penile cancer. The following tests and procedures may be used:

- **Physical Exam And History:** An exam of the body to check general signs of health, including checking the penis for signs of disease, such as lumps or anything else that seems unusual. A history of the patient's health habits and past illnesses and treatments will also be taken.

❖ **It's A Fact!!**

Human papillomavirus infection may increase the risk of developing penile cancer.

Circumcision may help prevent infection with the human papillomavirus (HPV). A circumcision is an operation in which the doctor removes part or all of the foreskin from the penis. Many boys are circumcised shortly after birth. Men who were not circumcised at birth may have a higher risk of developing penile cancer.

❖ **It's A Fact!!**
How Cancer Spreads

Cancer can spread through the body through:

- **Tissue:** Cancer invades the surrounding normal tissue.

- **The Lymph System:** Cancer invades the lymph system and travels through the lymph vessels to other places in the body.

- **The Blood:** Cancer invades the veins and capillaries and travels through the blood to other places in the body.

- **Biopsy:** The removal of cells or tissues so they can be viewed under a microscope by a pathologist to check for signs of cancer.

Prognosis

Certain factors affect prognosis and treatment options. The prognosis (chance of recovery) and treatment options depend on the stage of the cancer, the location and size of the tumor, and whether the cancer has just been diagnosed or has recurred (come back).

Stages Of Penile Cancer

After penile cancer has been diagnosed, tests are done to find out if cancer cells have spread within the penis or to other parts of the body. This process is called staging. The information gathered from the staging process determines the stage of the disease. It is important to know the stage in order to plan treatment.

The following stages are used for penile cancer:

Stage 0 (Carcinoma In Situ): In stage 0, abnormal cells or growths that look like warts are found on the surface of the skin of the penis. These abnormal cells or growths may become cancer and spread into nearby normal tissue. Stage 0 is also called carcinoma in situ.

Stage I: In stage I, cancer has formed and spread to connective tissue just under the skin of the penis. Cancer has not spread to lymph vessels or blood vessels. The tumor cells look a lot like normal cells under a microscope.

Stage II: In stage II, cancer has spread:

- to connective tissue just under the skin of the penis. Also, cancer has spread to lymph vessels or blood vessels or the tumor cells may look very different from normal cells under a microscope; or

- through connective tissue to erectile tissue (spongy tissue that fills with blood to make an erection); or

- beyond erectile tissue to the urethra.

Stage III: Stage III is divided into stage IIIa and stage IIIb. In stage IIIa, cancer has spread to one lymph node in the groin. Cancer has also spread:

- to connective tissue just under the skin of the penis. Also, cancer may have spread to lymph vessels or blood vessels or the tumor cells may look very different from normal cells under a microscope; or

- through connective tissue to erectile tissue (spongy tissue that fills with blood to make an erection); or

- beyond erectile tissue to the urethra.

In stage IIIb, cancer has spread to more than one lymph node on one side of the groin or to lymph nodes on both sides of the groin. Cancer has also spread:

- to connective tissue just under the skin of the penis. Also, cancer may have spread to lymph vessels or blood vessels or the tumor cells may look very different from normal cells under a microscope; or

- through connective tissue to erectile tissue (spongy tissue that fills with blood to make an erection); or

- beyond erectile tissue to the urethra.

Stage IV: In stage IV, cancer has spread:

- to tissues near the penis such as the prostate, and may have spread to lymph nodes in the groin or pelvis; or

- to one or more lymph nodes in the pelvis, or cancer has spread from the lymph nodes to the tissues around the lymph nodes; or

- to distant parts of the body.

❖ **It's A Fact!!**
Recurrent
Penile Cancer

Recurrent penile cancer is cancer that has recurred (come back) after it has been treated. The cancer may come back in the penis or in other parts of the body.

> ### ❧ It's A Fact!!
>
> Even if the doctor removes all the cancer that can be seen at the time of the surgery, some patients may be given chemotherapy or radiation therapy after surgery to kill any cancer cells that are left. Treatment given after the surgery, to lower the risk that the cancer will come back, is called adjuvant therapy.

Treatment Option Overview

Three types of standard treatment are used: surgery, radiation therapy, and chemotherapy.

Surgery

Surgery is the most common treatment for all stages of penile cancer. A doctor may remove the cancer using one of the following operations:

- **Mohs Microsurgery:** A procedure in which the tumor is cut from the skin in thin layers.

- **Laser Surgery:** A surgical procedure that uses a laser beam (a narrow beam of intense light) as a knife to make bloodless cuts in tissue or to remove a surface lesion such as a tumor.

- **Cryosurgery:** A treatment that uses an instrument to freeze and destroy abnormal tissue. This type of treatment is also called cryotherapy.

- **Circumcision:** Surgery to remove part or all of the foreskin of the penis.

- **Wide Local Excision:** Surgery to remove only the cancer and some normal tissue around it.

- **Amputation Of The Penis:** Surgery to remove part or all of the penis. If part of the penis is removed, it is a partial penectomy. If all of the penis is removed, it is a total penectomy.

Radiation Therapy

Radiation therapy is a cancer treatment that uses high-energy x-rays or other types of radiation to kill cancer cells or keep them from growing. There are two types of radiation therapy. External radiation therapy uses a machine outside the body to send radiation toward the cancer. Internal radiation therapy uses a radioactive substance sealed in needles, seeds, wires, or catheters that are placed directly into or near the cancer. The way the radiation therapy is given depends on the type and stage of the cancer being treated.

Chemotherapy

Chemotherapy is a cancer treatment that uses drugs to stop the growth of cancer cells, either by killing the cells or by stopping them from dividing. When chemotherapy is taken by mouth or injected into a vein or muscle, the drugs enter the bloodstream and can reach cancer cells throughout the body (systemic chemotherapy). When chemotherapy is placed directly onto the skin (topical chemotherapy) or into the cerebrospinal fluid, an organ, or a body cavity such as the abdomen, the drugs mainly affect cancer cells in those areas (regional chemotherapy). The way the chemotherapy is given depends on the type and stage of the cancer being treated.

♣ It's A Fact!!

New types of treatment are being tested in clinical trials. A treatment clinical trial is a research study meant to help improve current treatments or obtain information on new treatments for patients with cancer. When clinical trials show that a new treatment is better than the standard treatment, the new treatment may become the standard treatment. Patients may want to think about taking part in a clinical trial. Some clinical trials are open only to patients who have not started treatment.

Chapter 38

Testicular Exams

Medical exams, whether they're for school, a sport, or camp, are usually pretty straightforward. Many parts of the exam make sense to most guys: The scale is used to weigh you, the stethoscope is used to listen to your heartbeat.

But why does the doctor need to touch and feel your testicles? Isn't there a better, less embarrassing way to check things out?

When you are healthy and going for a physical exam, the doctor is interested in finding out specific things about your body and your health. He or she will check your height and weight, take your temperature, and take your blood pressure. The doctor will listen to your heart and lungs and will probably examine your eyes, ears, nose, and throat, and may also test your reflexes by tapping your knees and ankles. For all these parts of the exam, the doctor relies on tools and equipment to get the information that's needed.

However, for other parts of your body, the doctor's sense of touch and training are the key to knowing how things should feel. During the physical, the doctor will touch your belly to feel for any problems with your liver or spleen. He or

About This Chapter: Information in this chapter is from "Testicular Exams," April 2009, reprinted with permission from www.kidshealth.org. Copyright © 2009 The Nemours Foundation. This information was provided by KidsHealth, one of the largest resources online for medically reviewed health information written for parents, kids, and teens. For more articles like this one, visit www.KidsHealth.org, or www.TeensHealth.org.

she may also feel the lymph nodes in your neck, armpits, and groin to detect if there is any swelling, which can indicate an infection or other problem. And your doctor will also need to feel your testicles and the area around them to be sure they're developing properly and there are no problems.

♣ It's A Fact!!
Two possible problems that can affect teen guys are hernias and—rarely—testicular cancer.

Hernias

A hernia can occur when a part of the intestine pushes out from the abdomen and into the groin or scrotum (the sac of skin that the testicles hang in). Some people believe that this can only happen when a person lifts something heavy, but usually this isn't the case. Most hernias occur because of a weakness in the abdominal wall that the person was born with. If a piece of intestine becomes trapped in the scrotum, it can cut off the blood supply to the intestine and cause serious problems if the situation isn't quickly corrected.

A doctor is able to feel for a hernia by using his or her fingers to examine the area around the groin and testicles. The doctor may ask you to cough while pressing on or feeling the area. Sometimes, the hernia causes a bulge that the doctor can detect; if this happens, surgery almost always repairs the hernia completely.

Testicular Cancer

Although testicular cancer is unusual in teen guys (it occurs in three out of 100,000 guys between the ages of 15 and 19 in the United States), it is the second most common cancer seen during the teen years. It is the most common cancer in guys 20 to 34 years of age.

It's very important for your doctor to examine your testicles at least once a year. When doing so, your doctor will grasp one testicle at a time, rolling it gently between his or her thumb and first finger to feel for lumps and also checking whether the testicle is hardened or enlarged.

The doctor also will explain how to do testicular self-exams. Learning how to examine yourself at least once a month for any lumps or bumps on your testicles is very important. A tumor (growth or bump) on the testicles could be cancer. Knowing how your testicles feel when they're healthy will help you know when something feels different and possibly abnormal down there.

Finally, keep in mind that even though it might feel weird to have a doctor checking out your testicles, it's no big deal to him or her. Sometimes when a doctor is examining that area, you might get an erection—this is something you can't control. It's a normal reaction that happens frequently during genital exams on guys. If it happens, it won't upset or bother the doctor, so there's no need to feel embarrassed.

♣ It's A Fact!!

Noticing any new testicular lumps or bumps as soon as possible gives the best chances for survival and total cure if it turns out to be cancer.

Chapter 39

Testicular Trauma

Because the testicles are located within the scrotum, which hangs outside of the body, they do not have the protection of muscles and bones that most organs have. This makes it easier for the testicles to be struck, hit, kicked, or crushed. The following information should help explain why timely evaluation and proper management are critical for the best outcomes.

What happens under normal conditions?

As the producers of sperm and testosterone, the testicles are essential for reproduction and normal male hormones. But they are also prone to injuries that can leave damage to either the entire gland or essential parts of it.

Sperm cells are produced in the testicle and travel to the epididymis, a rubbery gland along the backside of the testicle that contains a single coiled tube formed by the merger of thousands of sperm-producing ducts originating inside the testicle. Sperm stop briefly in the epididymis to mature before exiting in semen through the vas deferens, a tube that connects with the urethra. Unlike the vas deferens, which is covered by a thick muscle wall, the epididymis has a coating that is both thin and fragile. As such, it is at higher risk for inflammation or injury.

❖ It's A Fact!!

Suspended in the scrotum, the skin pouch below
the penis, each testicle is surrounded by the tunica albuginea,
a tough, fibrous covering that encases and protects the delicate
gland tissue within it. Although tough, it can be torn or
"fractured" by a blunt or violent force.

What are the causes of testicular injury?

While testicular injuries can be from penetrating forces (e.g., stab wounds, gunshot wounds) or blunt forces (e.g., kick to the scrotum, baseball to the scrotum), they all have the potential of inflicting similar injuries: partial or complete ripping of the testicle as well as loss of the entire testicle. An injury sustained from a penetrating object such as a knife or bullet that punctures the scrotum may cause a minor scrape to the skin or major injury to the blood vessels to the testicle itself. An injury can also be caused by a direct blow—such as a kick or baseball to the groin—causing a tear in the covering of the testicle or injury to its blood vessels.

What are the symptoms of testicular injury?

While trauma to the testicle or scrotum usually produces severe pain as a first symptom, it can also result in actual physical injury to any of its contents. When the testicle's tough covering is torn or shattered, the blood leaks from the injury, stretching the normally elastic scrotum until it is tense. While this collection of blood can lead to infection, there also may be additional fertility problems due to the ultimate loss of a testicle or immune system problems that affect the remaining testicle. In severe cases of testicular injury, part or all of the injured testicle may need to be removed.

Considerable pain around the testicle may also be due to epididymitis, infection or inflammation of the epididymis. Because the epididymis, the lengthy coil alongside the testicle, is a very thin-walled gland it easily becomes red and swollen either by infection or injury. If left untreated, the condition rarely can lead to a loss of the testicle due to blockage of the blood supply to the testicle.

The symptoms mentioned above may indicate a very treatable, benign problem. But surprisingly, a substantial number of testicular tumors are discovered after minor injuries when men are more likely to carefully examine the testicles. Many men are not aware of the painless, solid lump, bulging from the smooth testicular covering until they have a reason to examine themselves. Do not make the mistake of many men who postpone medical care, thinking they are dealing with a simple bruise. This is a medical emergency! While testicular cancer caught early is generally curable, malignancies discovered late often require prolonged treatment involving surgery, radiation, and chemotherapy.

Men who suffer more than a minor injury to the scrotum should seek an evaluation by a urologist. Reasons to seek medical care include:

- any penetrating injury to the scrotum

- bruising and/or swelling of the scrotum

- difficulty urinating or blood in the urine

- fevers after testicular injury

How are testicular injuries treated?

A urologist can often determine the extent of injury to the testicle with a simple physical examination. After the urologist asks questions about how the injury occurred as well as other medical history questions, he or she will examine the contents of the scrotum. In doing so, the tough covering overlying the testicle can generally be easily felt as well as the narrow, soft epididymis. The structures that run into the testicle including the artery, vein, and vas deferens would then be felt to ensure that they are normal.

If everything appears normal, with no injury present, the urologist will probably prescribe pain medication such as acetaminophen or ibuprofen. A patient will also be advised to wear a jock strap, which provides good support for the scrotum.

If it is unclear if an injury has occurred, the urologist may request a scrotal ultrasound scan. Based on the same sonar sound waves that guide submarines, this device can safely and effectively image parts of the sac, including the testicle, epididymis, and spermatic cord, to examine the blood flow.

If any imaging study suggests testicular injury, the usual course of action is an operation where, under anesthesia, an incision is made in the scrotum and the entire contents are examined. If a tear of the testicle has occurred and the testicle can be repaired (if it has good blood supply and the remaining testicle has sufficient covering available), the urologist will usually repair the defect with stitches and then close the scrotum skin. In some cases, the urologist will leave a temporary plastic drain in the scrotum to drain blood and other fluids.

On occasion, an injury can be so severe that the testicle cannot be repaired. If this occurs, the urologist will remove the testicle. That does not mean the patient cannot father a child, however. If the patient's other testicle is normal, he should be able to impregnate his partner. Also, the patient's hormone levels should remain steady since only one testicle is required for either function.

If the patient's physical examination and ultrasound suggest that the injury has caused epididymitis, he will probably be treated without surgery, given an anti-inflammatory medication (such as ibuprofen) and encouraged again to wear a jock strap. If necessary, the urologist may also prescribe an antibiotic. It generally takes six to eight weeks for the swelling to subside. The patient may have to have several follow-up visits with the urologist to chart his progress. Further, if conservative measures (medications and jock strap) do not work, surgery may be required and the testicle may have to be removed.

❖ It's A Fact!!

Although no imaging test is 100 percent perfect, ultrasound is an attractive alternative because it is easy to perform, uses no X-rays, and clearly shows the physical structure of the scrotum. On rare occasions, the urologists may request an MRI, a more sophisticated imaging technique, if the ultrasound leaves more questions than answers.

Frequently Asked Questions

I have noticed pain in my scrotum and testicle but I do not remember any injury. What should I do?

There are many possible causes of scrotal or testicle pain including epididymitis, inflammation of the testicle, and problems with other parts of the scrotum. Whatever the source, you should be examined by a urologist, a specialist trained in such problems.

I was hit by a knee during a basketball game and have since noticed a new lump in my scrotum. It does not hurt but should I do anything about it?

Like many young men, you are probably examining yourself for the first time now that you have had a sporting injury. There is a good chance that the lump or "new" mass you have just felt is a normal part of the anatomy (your epididymis). But it could be an injury or even testicular cancer. Any new lump should be checked immediately by a trained urologist. With his/her expertise, a urologist will ease your mind and point you to swift and accurate treatment.

I'm 55 years old and noticed a lump in my scrotum after being hit in the groin during a pick-up game of baseball. Could this be testicular cancer or am I too old for that?

Testicular cancer can occur at any age, even though the most cases are between 15 and 35. Anyone with a new lump in the scrotum should see a urologist immediately. Often you will not need any further tests because the urologist can make a diagnosis with a physical examination. However, the urologist may also request an ultrasound. While some masses are not cancer (benign), many can be malignant. The good news, however, is that testicular cancer can be treated effectively if caught early. So do not be afraid to contact a urologist!

I noticed blood in my urine after being hit with a baseball. I do not feel any lumps. Should I still report this to my doctor?

Absolutely. Blood in the urine that is visible to the naked eye is almost always due to a urologic problem. You need to see a urologist immediately for evaluation to sort out the possibilities.

What can I do to prevent injury to my testicles?

There are many common-sense steps you can take to reduce your risk of testicular trauma. Wear a seat belt when driving a car. Make sure your clothes are tucked in and you are not exposing loose belts or other items to machinery that has exposed chains or belts. Wear a jock strap when playing sports. If the activity could produce severe contact (as in baseball, football, or hockey) use a hard cup to reduce the risk.

Chapter 40

Epididymitis And Orchitis

If you are a male and experiencing pain in the scrotum or testicle, then it might be attributed to epididymitis, orchitis, or a combination of the two. The information below will give you a head start in learning more about these conditions and aid you in your discussions with a urologist.

What are epididymitis, orchitis, and epididymo-orchitis?

Epididymitis is inflammation of the epididymis—the coiled tube that collects sperm from the testicle and passes it on to the vas deferens. There are two forms of this disease, acute and chronic. Acute epididymitis comes on suddenly with severe symptoms and subsides with treatment. Chronic epididymitis is a long-standing condition, usually of gradual onset, for which the symptoms can be improved with treatment but may not completely be eradicated. Most cases of epididymitis occur in adults.

Orchitis is inflammation of the testicle. It is almost always comes on suddenly and subsides with treatment. Chronic orchitis is not well defined, and instead is considered to be one of the many conditions related to chronic testicular pain (orchalgia).

Epididymo-orchitis is the sudden inflammation of both the epididymis and the testicle.

What are the causes of such conditions?

Acute epididymitis is usually caused by a bacterial infection. In children who haven't reached puberty, the infection usually starts in the bladder or kidney and then spreads to the testicle. This is often associated with a birth-related abnormality that predisposes to urinary tract infection. In sexually active men, the most common infection causing epididymitis is a sexually transmitted disease such as gonorrhea or chlamydia infection. These infections start in the urethra, causing urethritis, which can then move into the testicle. In men over 40 years of age, the most common cause is bacteria from the urinary tract. Other causes can include: bladder outlet obstruction due to enlargement of the prostate; partial blockage of the urethra; bacterial prostatitis (an infection of the prostate gland); or recent catheterization of the urethra. In any of these cases, the original infection may not cause symptoms, and the first sign of a problem may be epididymitis. Bacterial epididymitis rarely occurs when a bacterial infection spreads from the bloodstream into the epididymis, although this is the typical way that tuberculosis infection can involve the epididymis.

Chronic epididymitis may develop after several episodes of acute epididymitis that do not subside, but also can occur without any symptomatic episodes of acute epididymitis or prior infection—in which case the cause is unknown.

✤ It's A Fact!!

Epididymitis is occasionally due to causes other than infection. Chemical epididymitis occurs when sterile urine flows backward from the urethra to the epididymis, which most commonly occurs with heavy lifting or straining. The urine causes inflammation without infection. The drug amiodarone also can cause a non-infectious epididymitis, and there are other cases of non-infectious epididymitis without known cause.

In most cases of acute orchitis, the testicle is inflamed due to the spread of a bacterial infection from the epididymis, and therefore "epididymo-orchitis" is the correct term. Although orchitis without epididymitis can occur from a bacterial infection, orchitis without epididymitis usually results from an infection related to the mumps virus (or other virus infections). "Mumps orchitis" occurs in approximately one-third of males who contract mumps after puberty.

Acute epididymo-orchitis is usually a primary bacterial or rarely a tuberculous infection of the epididymis that has spread to the testicle to involve both structures. Rarely, it can start in the testicle and spread to the epididymis. Mumps orchitis does not spread to the epididymis.

What are the symptoms and how are they diagnosed?

Acute Epididymitis And Acute Epididymo-Orchitis: Symptoms occur not only from the local infection, but also from the original source of the infection. Common symptoms from the original source of the infection include: urethral discharge and urethral pain or itching (from urethritis); pelvic pain and urinary frequency, urgency, or painful/burning urination (from infection of the bladder, called cystitis); fever, perineal pain, urinary frequency, urinary urgency, or painful/burning urination (from infection of the prostate, called prostatitis); fever and flank pain (from infection of the kidney, called pyelonephritis). In some cases, pain in the scrotum from the local infection is the only noticeable symptom. The pain starts at the back of one testicle but can soon spread to the entire testicle, the scrotum, and occasionally the groin. Swelling, tenderness, redness, firmness, and warmth of the skin may also accompany the pain. The entire scrotum can swell up with fluid (hydrocele). To make the diagnosis, the doctor will ask you about your medical history and examine you. The doctor may test a urine sample and look at it under the microscope to assess for bacterial infection, culture a urine sample as a more definitive way to see if there is bacterial infection, or examine a swab obtained from the urethra (if urethritis is suggested by your symptoms).

Chronic Epididymitis: The pain occurs only in the scrotal contents, and is less severe and more localized than acute epididymitis. Swelling, tenderness, redness, and warmth of the skin do not occur. Additional tests may be used as for acute epididymitis, but are less frequently required. In acute epididymitis the urine is usually infected, whereas in chronic epididymitis it is usually not.

Acute Orchitis: During the acute phase of mumps orchitis, symptoms include pain of varying severity, tenderness, and swelling. The parotiditis (swelling of facial glands) of mumps usually precedes orchitis by three to seven days. Isolated orchitis from bacterial infection has the same symptoms of acute epididymitis or epididymo-orchitis.

> **❖ It's A Fact!!**
> If your pain came on very suddenly and severely, then an ultrasound, which is a non-invasive test that uses sound waves to look at the epididymis and measure blood flow, might be used to distinguish epididymitis from another condition called testicular torsion. This is managed very differently than epididymitis, so making the distinction is very important. Tuberculous epididymitis presents in the same way, although chemical and amiodarone epididymitis are less severe.

What are the treatment options?

Acute Epididymitis And Acute Epididymo-Orchitis: Treatment in cases suspected to be from bacteria (most) includes at least two weeks of antibiotics. Most cases can be treated with oral antibiotics as an outpatient. Your doctor can choose one of several, including: doxycycline, azithromycin, ofloxacin, ciprofloxacin, levofloxacin, or trimethoprim-sulfamethoxazole. Tuberculous epididymitis is treated with anti-tuberculous medications, although in many cases surgical removal of the testicle (orchiectomy, which includes removal of the epididymis) is required because the damage is so severe. Cases of severe infection, with intractable pain, vomiting, very high fever, or overall severe illness, may require admission to the hospital. Aside from treatment of amidarone epididymitis by reducing the dose or stopping the drug, there is no specific therapy for non-infectious epididymitis. General therapy for epididymitis includes bed rest for one to two days combined with elevation of the scrotum. The aim is to get the inflamed epididymis above the level of the heart. This improves blood flow out of the testicle, which promotes more rapid healing and reduces swelling and discomfort. Intermittent application of ice might also be of assistance and, in cases due to infection, intake of plenty of fluids.

Chronic Epididymitis: Primary therapy is with medications and other treatments directed towards reducing the discomfort. Non-steroidal anti-inflammatory medications and local application of heat are the mainstays of treatment. If symptoms persist, your physician may recommend other medications to alter the perception of pain in the area, or might refer you to a specialist in pain management. If all else fails the epididymis can be surgically removed (epididymectomy) while leaving the testicle in place.

Acute Orchitis: There is no specific treatment for acute mumps orchitis. In cases of bacterial infection, treatment is as for acute epididymitis and acute epididymo-orchitis.

What can be expected after treatment?

Acute Epididymitis And Acute Epididymo-Orchitis: In the typical infectious case, it will take two to three days for you to notice improvement. If the redness does not subside and you do not start to feel better by that time, contact your physician. Complete resolution of symptoms will take longer. Discomfort can persist until the entire course of antibiotics is completed, and the firmness and swelling can takes months to resolve. Following the instructions to stay at bed rest with scrotal elevation for the first one to two days will help speed recovery. You should follow up with your physician after treatment. In cases of tuberculous epididymitis that do not require orchiectomy, it takes months to resolve on medications, and there will likely be some shrinking of the testicle. Amidarone epididymitis improves after reducing the dose or stopping the drug, without any residual problems. Chemical epididymitis also resolves completely.

❖ **It's A Fact!!**
Nonsteroidal anti-inflammatory drugs such as ibuprofen or naproxen are useful since they not only relieve pain but also reduce the inflammation that is the cause of the pain.

Chronic Epididymitis: Treatment is ongoing, and not curative. You may need to take medications for years, or until the symptoms resolve spontaneously. If epididymectomy is performed, relief of symptoms occurs in three out of four patients after a few weeks for surgical recovery. If surgery has not resolved your symptoms, then your doctor will try medical therapy again.

Acute Orchitis: Following the acute phase of mumps orchitis, the pain resolves but there is often atrophy of the testicle.

Frequently Asked Questions

What if the swelling and pain do not get better after the first three days of antibiotics?

Most cases of acute epididymitis or epididymo-orchitis are treated well by antibiotics, but in some cases a different antibiotic needs to be used. Tuberculous epididymitis should also be considered when symptoms do not resolve appropriately. On occasion, surgery needs to be performed. If an abscess (pocket of pus) has formed, antibiotics alone are rarely sufficient and surgery to drain the abscess or remove part or all of the epididymis and testicle might be required. Other complications that might require surgery include testicular infarction (death of the testicle due to destruction of the blood vessels) and cutaneous fistula (infection that continues to drain out through the skin).

Can I pass the infection to my sexual partner?

If the acute epididymitis or epididymo-orchitis is from a sexually transmitted disease (usually in sexually active men under 40 years of age), then your sexual partner needs to be treated as well since the infection can be passed back and forth through sexual contact. The urinary tract bacteria that cause other cases of epididymitis or epididymo-orchitis are not sexually transmitted. Treatment of your partner is not required, and there is no risk of infecting your partner.

Will the ability to father children be reduced?

The atrophy associated with mumps orchitis and tuberculous epididymitis is associated with reduced production of sperm in the affected testicle in some cases. After an episode of acute epididymitis or epididymo-orchitis there can rarely be blockage of the epididymis, which would reduce delivery of sperm from that testicle. In any of these cases, if the other testicle is unaffected then most men are able to father a child normally.

Will hormone production by the testicle be affected?

The ability of the affected testicle to produce testosterone is lost in some men with atrophy associated with mumps orchitis and tuberculous epididymitis. The rare epididymal blockage that occurs after acute epididymitis or epididymo-orchitis does not affect hormone production.

Do epididymal or testicular infections lead to cancer?

There is no association of these infections with cancer.

Chapter 41

Hypogonadism

Hypogonadism is when the sex glands produce little or no hormones. In men, these glands (gonads) are the testes; in women, they are the ovaries.

Causes

The cause of hypogonadism may be "primary" or "central." In primary hypogonadism, the ovaries or testes themselves do not function properly. Some causes of primary hypogonadism include:

- certain autoimmune disorders
- genetic and developmental disorders
- infection
- liver and kidney disease
- radiation
- surgery

In central hypogonadism, the centers in the brain that control the gonads (hypothalamus and pituitary) do not function properly. Some causes of central hypogonadism include:

About This Chapter: Information in this chapter is from "Hypogonadism," © 2010 A.D.A.M., Inc. Reprinted with permission.

- bleeding

- genetic problems

- infections

- nutritional deficiencies

- iron excess (hemochromatosis)

- radiation

- rapid, significant weight loss

- surgery

- trauma

- tumors

> ✣ **It's A Fact!!**
> The most common genetic disorders that cause primary hypogonadism are Turner syndrome (in women) and Klinefelter syndrome (in men).

Symptoms

In girls, hypogonadism during childhood will result in lack of menstruation and breast development and short height. If hypogonadism occurs after puberty, symptoms include loss of menstruation, low libido, hot flashes, and loss of body hair.

In boys, hypogonadism in childhood results in lack of muscle and beard development and growth problems. In men the usual complaints are sexual dysfunction, decreased beard and body hair, breast enlargement, and muscle loss.

If a brain tumor is present (central hypogonadism), there may be headaches or visual loss, or symptoms of other hormonal deficiencies (such as hypothyroidism). In the case of the most common pituitary tumor, prolactinoma, there may be a milky breast discharge. People with anorexia nervosa (excessive dieting to the point of starvation) and those who undergo rapid, extreme weight loss, as seen after gastric bypass surgery, also may have central hypogonadism.

Exams And Tests

Tests may be done that check estrogen level (women) and testosterone level (men) as well as FSH level and LH level, the pituitary hormones that stimulate the gonads. Other tests may include a thyroid level; sperm count;

prolactin level (milk hormone); blood tests for anemia, chemistries, and iron; and genetic analysis.

Sometimes imaging is necessary, such as a sonogram of the ovaries. If pituitary disease is suspected, an MRI or CT scan of the brain may be done.

Treatment

Hormone-based medicines are available for men and women. Estrogen comes in the form of a patch or pill. Testosterone can be given by using a patch, a product soaked in by the gums, a gel, or by injection.

For women who have not had their uterus removed, combination treatment with estrogen and progesterone is often recommended to decrease the chances of developing endometrial cancer. In addition, low dose testosterone can be added for women with hypogonadism who have a low sex drive.

In some women, injections or pills can be used to stimulate ovulation. Injections of pituitary hormone may be used to help male patients produce sperm. In others, surgery and radiation therapy may be needed.

Outlook (Prognosis)

Many forms of hypogonadism are potentially treatable and have a good prognosis.

Possible Complications

In women, hypogonadism may cause infertility. Menopause is a form of hypogonadism that occurs naturally and can cause hot flashes, vaginal dryness, and irritability as a woman's estrogen levels fall. The risk of osteoporosis and heart disease increase after menopause.

♣ It's A Fact!!

A genetic cause of central hypogonadism that also produces an inability to smell is Kallmann syndrome (males). The most common tumors affecting the pituitary area are craniopharyngioma (in children) and prolactinoma (in adults).

Some women with hypogonadism opt to take estrogen therapy, particularly those who have early menopause (premature ovarian failure). However, there is a small but significant increase in risk for breast cancer and possibly heart disease with use of hormone therapy for treatment of menopause symptoms.

In men, hypogonadism results in loss of sex drive and may cause weakness, impotence, infertility, and osteoporosis. Men normally experience some decline in testosterone as they age, but it is not as dramatic or steep as the decline in sex hormones experienced by women.

When To Contact A Medical Professional

Consult with your doctor if you notice loss of menstruation, breast discharge, problems getting pregnant, hot flashes (women), impotence, loss of body hair, weakness, breast enlargement (men), or problems with your sex drive. Both men and women should call their health care providers if headaches or visual problems occur.

Prevention

Maintain normal body weight and healthy eating habits to prevent anorexia nervosa. Other causes may not be preventable.

Chapter 42

Testicular Cancer

Testicular cancer is a disease in which cells become malignant (cancerous) in one or both testicles.

The testicles (also called testes or gonads) are a pair of male sex glands. They produce and store sperm and are the main source of testosterone (male hormones) in men. These hormones control the development of the reproductive organs and other male physical characteristics. The testicles are located under the penis in a sac-like pouch called the scrotum.

Based on the characteristics of the cells in the tumor, testicular cancers are classified as seminomas or nonseminomas. Other types of cancer that arise in the testicles are rare and are not described here. Seminomas may be one of three types: classic, anaplastic, or spermatocytic. Types of nonseminomas include choriocarcinoma, embryonal carcinoma, teratoma, and yolk sac tumors. Testicular tumors may contain both seminoma and nonseminoma cells.

About This Chapter: This chapter begins with information from "Testicular Cancer: Questions and Answers," a publication on the website of the National Cancer Institute (http://www.cancer.gov), May 2005. Reviewed by David A. Cooke, MD, FACP, October 2010. The chapter concludes with "How to Do a Testicular Self Examination," © 2009 Testicular Cancer Resource Center (http://tcrc.acor.org). Reprinted with permission.

Risk Factors

The exact causes of testicular cancer are not known. However, studies have shown that several factors increase a man's chance of developing this disease.

- **Undescended Testicle (Cryptorchidism):** Normally, the testicles descend from inside the abdomen into the scrotum before birth. The risk of testicular cancer is increased in males with a testicle that does not move down into the scrotum. This risk does not change even after surgery to move the testicle into the scrotum. The increased risk applies to both testicles.

- **Congenital Abnormalities:** Men born with abnormalities of the testicles, penis, or kidneys, as well as those with inguinal hernia (hernia in the groin area, where the thigh meets the abdomen), may be at increased risk.

- **History Of Testicular Cancer:** Men who have had testicular cancer are at increased risk of developing cancer in the other testicle.

- **Family History Of Testicular Cancer:** The risk for testicular cancer is greater in men whose brother or father has had the disease.

♣ It's A Fact!!

Testicular cancer accounts for only one percent of all cancers in men in the United States. About 8,000 men are diagnosed with testicular cancer, and about 390 men die of this disease each year. Testicular cancer occurs most often in men between the ages of 20 and 39, and is the most common form of cancer in men between the ages of 15 and 34. It is most common in white men, especially those of Scandinavian descent. The testicular cancer rate has more than doubled among white men in the past 40 years, but has only recently begun to increase among black men. The reason for the racial differences in incidence is not known.

Source: National Cancer Institute, May 2005. Reviewed by David A. Cooke, MD, FACP, October 2010.

Symptoms

Most testicular cancers are found by men themselves. Also, doctors generally examine the testicles during routine physical exams. Between regular checkups, if a man notices anything unusual about his testicles, he should talk with his doctor. Men should see a doctor if they notice any of the following symptoms:

• A painless lump or swelling in a testicle

• Pain or discomfort in a testicle or in the scrotum

• Any enlargement of a testicle or change in the way it feels

• A feeling of heaviness in the scrotum

• A dull ache in the lower abdomen, back, or groin

• A sudden collection of fluid in the scrotum

These symptoms can be caused by cancer or by other conditions. It is important to see a doctor to determine the cause of any of these symptoms.

Diagnosis

To help find the cause of symptoms, the doctor evaluates a man's general health. The doctor also performs a physical exam and may order laboratory and diagnostic tests. These tests include:

• **Blood Tests That Measure The Levels Of Tumor Markers:** Tumor markers are substances often found in higher-than-normal amounts when cancer is present. Tumor markers such as alpha-fetoprotein (AFP), Beta-human chorionic gonadotropin (ßHCG), and lactate dehydrogenase (LDH) may suggest the presence of a testicular tumor, even if it is too small to be detected by physical exams or imaging tests.

• **Ultrasound:** This is a test in which high-frequency sound waves are bounced off internal organs and tissues. Their echoes produce a picture called a sonogram. Ultrasound of the scrotum can show the presence and size of a mass in the testicle. It is also helpful in ruling out other conditions, such as swelling due to infection or a collection of fluid unrelated to cancer.

- **Biopsy:** This is a microscopic examination of testicular tissue by a pathologist to determine whether cancer is present. In nearly all cases of suspected cancer, the entire affected testicle is removed through an incision in the groin. This procedure is called radical inguinal orchiectomy. In rare cases (for example, when a man has only one testicle), the surgeon performs an inguinal biopsy, removing a sample of tissue from the testicle through an incision in the groin and proceeding with orchiectomy only if the pathologist finds cancer cells. (The surgeon does not cut through the scrotum to remove tissue. If the problem is cancer, this procedure could cause the disease to spread.)

If testicular cancer is found, more tests are needed to find out if the cancer has spread from the testicle to other parts of the body. Determining the stage (extent) of the disease helps the doctor to plan appropriate treatment.

Treatment

Although the incidence of testicular cancer has risen in recent years, more than 95 percent of cases can be cured. Treatment is more likely to be successful when testicular cancer is found early. In addition, treatment can often be less aggressive and may cause fewer side effects.

❖ It's A Fact!!

Men with testicular cancer should discuss their concerns about sexual function and fertility with their doctor. It is important to know that men with testicular cancer often have fertility problems even before their cancer is treated. If a man has pre-existing fertility problems, or if he is to have treatment that might lead to infertility, he may want to ask the doctor about sperm banking (freezing sperm before treatment for use in the future). This procedure allows some men to have children even if the treatment causes loss of fertility.

Source: National Cancer Institute, May 2005. Reviewed by David A. Cooke, MD, FACP, October 2010.

Most men with testicular cancer can be cured with surgery, radiation therapy, and/or chemotherapy. The side effects depend on the type of treatment and may be different for each person.

Seminomas and nonseminomas grow and spread differently and are treated differently. Nonseminomas tend to grow and spread more quickly; seminomas are more sensitive to radiation. If the tumor contains both seminoma and nonseminoma cells, it is treated as a nonseminoma. Treatment also depends on the stage of the cancer, the patient's age and general health, and other factors. Treatment is often provided by a team of specialists, which may include a surgeon, a medical oncologist, and a radiation oncologist.

Follow-Up Treatment

Regular follow-up exams are extremely important for men who have been treated for testicular cancer. Like all cancers, testicular cancer can recur (come back). Men who have had testicular cancer should see their doctor regularly and should report any unusual symptoms right away. Follow-up varies for different types and stages of testicular cancer. Generally, patients are checked frequently by their doctor and have regular blood tests to measure tumor marker levels. They also have regular x-rays and computed tomography, also called CT scans or CAT scans (detailed pictures of areas inside the body created by a computer linked to an x-ray machine). Men who have had testicular cancer have an increased likelihood of developing cancer in the remaining testicle. Patients treated with chemotherapy may have an increased risk of certain types of leukemia, as well as other types of cancer. Regular follow-up care ensures that changes in health are discussed and that problems are treated as soon as possible.

How To Do A Testicular Self-Examination

For men over the age of 14, a monthly self-exam of the testicles is an effective way of becoming familiar with this area of the body and thus enabling the detection of testicular cancer at an early—and very curable—stage. Why do you need to do it monthly? Because the point of the self-exam is not to find something wrong today. The point is to learn what everything feels like when things are normal, and to check back every month to make sure that nothing has changed. If something HAS changed, you will know it and you can do something about it.

Here is how to do the self-exam:

- If possible, stand in front of a mirror. Check for any swelling on the scrotal skin.

- Examine each testicle with both hands. Place the index and middle fingers under the testicle with the thumbs placed on top. Roll the testicle gently between the thumbs and fingers—you shouldn't feel any pain when doing the exam. Don't be alarmed if one testicle seems slightly larger than the other, that's normal.

- Find the epididymis, the soft, tubelike structure behind the testicle that collects and carries sperm. If you are familiar with this structure, you won't mistake it for a suspicious lump. Cancerous lumps usually are found on the sides of the testicle but can also show up on the front. Lumps on or attached to the epididymis are not cancerous.

- If you find a lump on your testicle or any of the other signs of testicular cancer listed below, see a doctor, preferably a urologist, right away. The abnormality may not be cancer, but if it is testicular cancer, it will spread if it is not stopped by treatment. Even if it is something else like an infection, you are still going to need to see a doctor. Waiting and hoping will not fix anything. Please note that free-floating lumps in the scrotum that are not attached in any way to a testicle are not testicular cancer. When in doubt, get it checked out—if only for peace of mind!

Other signs of testicular cancer to keep in mind are:

- any enlargement of a testicle

- a significant loss of size in one of the testicles

- a feeling of heaviness in the scrotum

- a dull ache in the lower abdomen or in the groin

- a sudden collection of fluid in the scrotum

- pain or discomfort in a testicle or in the scrotum

- enlargement or tenderness of the breasts

✔ **Quick Tip**

The testicular self-exam is best performed after a warm bath or shower. (Heat relaxes the scrotum, making it easier to spot anything abnormal.)

Source: © 2009 Testicular Cancer Resource Center.

I hesitate to mention the following list, since anything out of the ordinary down there should prompt a visit to the doctor, but you should be aware that the following symptoms are not normally signs of testicular cancer:

- a pimple, ingrown hair or rash on the scrotal skin

- a free-floating lump in the scrotum, seemingly not attached to anything

- a lump on the epidiymis or tubes coming from the testicle that kind of feels like a third testicle

- pain or burning during urination

- blood in the urine or semen

✔ Quick Tip

Remember, only a physician can make a positive diagnosis.

For that matter, only a physician can make a negative diagnosis too. If you think something feels strange, go see the doctor!

Finally, embarrassment is a poor excuse for not having any problem examined by a doctor. If you think there is something wrong or something has changed, please see your doctor!

Source: © 2009 Testicular Cancer Resource Center.

Chapter 43

Klinefelter Syndrome

What is Klinefelter syndrome?

Klinefelter syndrome is a condition that occurs in men as a result of an extra X chromosome. The most common symptom is infertility.

Humans have 46 chromosomes, which contain all of a person's genes and DNA. Two of these chromosomes, the sex chromosomes, determine a person's gender. Both of the sex chromosomes in females are called X chromosomes. (This is written as XX.) Males have an X and a Y chromosome (written as XY). The two sex chromosomes help a person develop fertility and the sexual characteristics of their gender.

Most often, Klinefelter syndrome is the result of one extra X (written as XXY). Occasionally, variations of the XXY chromosome count may occur, the most common being the XY/XXY mosaic. In this variation, some of the cells in the male's body have an additional X chromosome, and the rest have the normal XY chromosome count. The percentage of cells containing the extra chromosome varies from case to case. In some instances, XY/XXY mosaics may have enough normally functioning cells in the testes to allow the male to father children.

About This Chapter: Information in this chapter is from "Learning About Klinefelter Syndrome," a publication of the National Human Genome Research Institute, National Institutes of Health, October 2009.

What are the symptoms of Klinefelter syndrome?

Males who have Klinefelter syndrome may have the following symptoms: small, firm testes; a small penis; sparse pubic, armpit, and facial hair; enlarged breasts (called gynecomastia); tall stature; and abnormal body proportions (long legs, short trunk).

School-age children may be diagnosed if they are referred to a doctor to evaluate learning disabilities. The diagnosis may also be considered in the adolescent male when puberty is not progressing as expected. Adult males may come to the doctor because of infertility.

✤ It's A Fact!!

Klinefelter syndrome is found in about one out of every 500–1,000 newborn males. The additional sex chromosome results from a random error during the formation of the egg or sperm. About half of the time the error occurs in the formation of sperm, while the remainder are due to errors in egg development. Women who have pregnancies after age 35 have a slightly increased chance of having a boy with this syndrome.

Klinefelter syndrome is associated with an increased risk for breast cancer, a rare tumor called extragonadal germ cell tumor, lung disease, varicose veins, and osteoporosis. Men who have Klinefelter syndrome also have an increased risk for autoimmune disorders such as lupus, rheumatoid arthritis, and Sjogren's syndrome.

How is Klinefelter syndrome diagnosed?

A chromosomal analysis (karyotype) is used to confirm the diagnosis. In this procedure, a small blood sample is drawn. White blood cells are then separated from the sample, mixed with tissue culture medium, incubated, and checked for chromosomal abnormalities, such as an extra X chromosome.

The chromosome analysis looks at a number of cells, usually at least 20, which allows for the diagnosis of genetic conditions in both the full and mosaic state. In some cases, low-level mosaicism may be missed. However, if mosaicism is suspected (based on hormone levels, sperm counts, or physical characteristics), additional cells can be analyzed from within the same blood draw.

How is Klinefelter syndrome treated?

Testosterone therapy is used to increase strength, promote muscular development, grow body hair, improve mood and self-esteem, increase energy, and improve concentration.

Most men who have Klinefelter syndrome can expect to have a normal and productive life. Early diagnosis, in conjunction with educational interventions, medical management, and strong social support, will optimize each individual's potential in adulthood.

❖ It's A Fact!!

Most men who have Klinefelter syndrome are not able to father children. However, some men with an extra X chromosome have fathered healthy offspring, sometimes with the help of infertility specialists.

Chapter 44

Gynecomastia

Gynecomastia is the development of abnormally large breasts in males. It is related to the excess growth of breast tissue, rather than excess fat tissue.

Considerations

The condition may occur in one or both breasts and begins as a small lump beneath the nipple, which may be tender. The breasts often enlarge unevenly. Gynecomastia during puberty is not uncommon and usually goes away over a period of months.

In newborns, breast development may be associated with milk flow (galactorrhea). This condition usually lasts for a couple of weeks, but in rare cases may last until the child is two years old.

Causes

Androgens are hormones that create male characteristics, such as hair growth, muscle size, and a deep voice. Estrogens are hormones that create female characteristics. All men have both androgens and estrogens.

Changes in the levels of these hormones, or in how the body uses or responds to these hormones can cause enlarged breasts in men.

About This Chapter: Information in this chapter is from "Gynecomastia," © 2010 A.D.A.M., Inc. Reprinted with permission.

Other causes include:

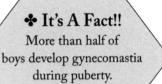

• aging

• cancer chemotherapy

• chronic liver disease

• exposure to anabolic steroid hormones

• exposure to estrogen hormone

• kidney failure and dialysis

• marijuana use

• hormone treatment for prostate cancer

• radiation treatment of the testicles

• side effects of some medications (ketoconazole, spironolactone, metronidazole, cimetidine (Tagamet))

• testosterone (male hormone) deficiency

Rare causes include:

• genetic defects

• overactive thyroid

• tumors

Breast cancer in men is rare. Signs that may suggest breast cancer include:

• one-sided breast growth

• firm or hard breast lump that feels like it is attached to the tissue

• skin ulcer over the breast

• bloody discharge from the nipple

Home Care

Apply cold compresses and use analgesics as your health care provider recommends if swollen breasts are also tender.

Other tips include:

- Stop taking all recreational drugs, such as marijuana.

- Stop taking all nutritional supplements or any drugs you are taking for bodybuilding.

When To Contact A Medical Professional

Call your health care provider if:

- you have recent swelling, pain, or enlargement in one or both breasts

- there is dark or bloody discharge from the nipples

- there is a skin sore or ulcer over the breast

- a breast lump feels hard or firm

Note: Gynecomastia in children who have not yet reached puberty should always be checked by a health care provider.

What To Expect At Your Office Visit

Your health care provider will take a medical history and perform a physical examination.

Medical history questions may include:

- Is one or both breasts involved?

- What is the age and gender of the patient?

- What medications is the person taking?

- How long has gynecomastia been present?

- Is the gynecomastia staying the same, getting better, or getting worse?

- What other symptoms are present?

Testing may not be necessary, but the following tests may be done to rule out certain diseases:

- blood hormone level tests

- breast ultrasound

- liver and kidney function studies

- mammogram

Intervention: If an underlying condition is found, it is treated. Your physician should consider all medications that may be causing the problem. Gynecomastia during puberty usually goes away on its own.

❖ It's A Fact!!

Breast enlargement that is extreme, uneven, or does not go away may be embarrassing for an adolescent boy. Treatments that may be used in rare situations are:

- hormone treatment that blocks the effects of estrogens

- breast reduction surgery

Part Five

Pregnancy Prevention

Chapter 45

Teen Pregnancy Facts

Following Decade-Long Decline, U.S. Teen Pregnancy Rate Increases As Both Births And Abortions Rise

Gap Between Blacks And Hispanics Has Closed, But Rates Among Both Groups Remain Significantly Higher Than Among Non-Hispanic Whites

For the first time in more than a decade, the nation's teen pregnancy rate rose 3% in 2006, reflecting increases in teen birth and abortion rates of 4% and 1%, respectively.

These new data from the Guttmacher Institute are especially noteworthy because they provide the first documentation of what experts have suspected for several years, based on trends in teens' contraceptive use—that the overall teen pregnancy rate would increase in the mid-2000s following steep declines in the 1990s and a subsequent plateau in the early 2000s. The significant drop

About This Chapter: Information in this chapter is from the Guttmacher Institute, "Following decade-long decline, U.S. teen pregnancy rate increases as both births and abortions rise," news release, New York: Guttmacher Institute, January 26, 2010, http://www.guttmacher.org/media/nr/2010/01/26/index.html, accessed September 2010. The chapter also includes excerpts from "U.S. Teenage Birth Rate Resumes Decline," National Center for Health Statistics, Centers for Disease Control and Prevention, February 2011.

in teen pregnancy rates in the 1990s was overwhelmingly the result of more and better use of contraceptives among sexually active teens. However, this decline started to stall out in the early 2000s, at the same time that sex education programs aimed exclusively at promoting abstinence—and prohibited by law from discussing the benefits of contraception—became increasingly widespread and teens' use of contraceptives declined.

"After more than a decade of progress, this reversal is deeply troubling," says Heather Boonstra, Guttmacher Institute senior public policy associate. "It coincides with an increase in rigid abstinence-only-until-marriage programs, which received major funding boosts under the Bush administration. A strong body of research shows that these programs do not work. Fortunately, the heyday of this failed experiment has come to an end with the enactment of a new teen pregnancy prevention initiative that ensures that programs will be age-appropriate, medically accurate and, most importantly, based on research demonstrating their effectiveness."

The teen pregnancy rate declined 41% between its peak, in 1990 (116.9 pregnancies per 1,000 women aged 15–19), and 2005 (69.5 per 1,000). Teen birth and abortion rates also declined, with births dropping 35% between 1991 and 2005 and teen abortion declining 56% between its peak, in 1988, and 2005. But all three trends reversed in 2006. In that year, there were 71.5 pregnancies per 1,000 women aged 15–19. Put another way, about 7% of teen girls became pregnant in 2006.

Just as the long-term declines in teen pregnancy occurred among all racial and ethnic groups through 2005, the reversal in 2006 also involved all demographic groups:

- Among black teens, the pregnancy rate declined by 45% (from 223.8 per 1,000 in 1990 to 122.7 in 2005), before increasing to 126.3 in 2006.

- Among Hispanic teens, the pregnancy rate decreased by 26% (from 169.7 per 1,000 in 1992 to 124.9 in 2005), before rising to 126.6 in 2006.

- Among non-Hispanic white teens, the pregnancy rate declined 50% (from 86.6 per 1,000 in 1990 to 43.3 per 1,000 in 2005), before increasing to 44.0 in 2006.

Because the decline among black teens was so much greater than that among Hispanics, the long-standing gap between the two groups has disappeared. However, the gap between white teens and teens of color is as large as ever.

State-level data are not yet available for 2006, but varied widely in 2005. The highest pregnancy rates were in New Mexico (93 per 1,000 women 15–19), Nevada (90), Arizona (89), Texas (88), and Mississippi (85), and the lowest rates were in New Hampshire (33), Vermont (40), Maine (48), Minnesota (47), and North Dakota (46). Teen pregnancy rates declined in every state between 1988 and 2000, and in every state except North Dakota between 2000 and 2005.

"It is too soon to tell whether the increase in the teen pregnancy rate between 2005 and 2006 is a short term fluctuation, a more lasting stabilization or the beginning of a significant new trend, any of which would be of great concern," says Lawrence Finer, Guttmacher's director of domestic research. "Either way, it is clearly time to redouble our efforts to make sure our young people have the information, interpersonal skills, and health services they need to prevent unwanted pregnancies and to become sexually healthy adults."

U.S. Teenage Birth Rate Resumes Decline: New Report Updates Trends In Teen Pregnancy

The U.S. teen birth rate fell by more than one-third from 1991 through 2005, but then increased by 5 percent over two consecutive years. Data for 2008 and 2009, however, indicate that the long-term downward trend has resumed. Although the recent declines have been widespread by age, race and

---

❖ It's A Fact!!

Teenage childbearing has been the subject of long-standing concern among the public and policy makers. Teenagers who give birth are much more likely to deliver a low birthweight or preterm infant than older women, and their babies are at elevated risk of dying in infancy. The annual public costs associated with teen childbearing have been estimated at $9.1 billion.

Source: Centers for Disease Control and Prevention, February 2011.

ethnicity, and state, large disparities nevertheless persist in these characteristics. The most current data available from the National Vital Statistics System are used to illustrate trends and variations through 2009.

- The teenage birth rate declined 8 percent in the United States from 2007 through 2009, reaching a historic low (the lowest it has ever been in the nearly 70 years for which national data are available) at 39.1 births per 1,000 teens aged 15–19 years.

- The number of births to teenagers aged 15–19 in 2009 fell to 409,840, the fewest since 1946 and 36 percent fewer than in 1970 (644,708), the historic high point.

- Rates fell significantly for teenagers in all age groups and for all racial and ethnic groups.

- Teenage birth rates for each age group and for nearly all race and Hispanic origin groups in 2009 were at the lowest levels ever reported in the United States.

- Birth rates for teens aged 15–17 dropped in 31 states from 2007 through 2009; rates for older teenagers aged 18–19 declined significantly in 45 states during this period.

While the U.S. teenage birth rate fell 37 percent from 1991 through 2009, it still remains the highest among industrialized countries. The recent trend marks a resumption of the long-term decline in teenage childbearing that started in 1991. Previous studies have suggested that these declines reflected the impact of strong teenage pregnancy prevention messages that accompanied a variety of public and private efforts to focus teenagers' attention on the importance of avoiding pregnancy. Data from several cycles of the National Survey of Family Growth (NSFG) conducted by the Centers for Disease Control and Prevention's National Center for Health Statistics (CDC/NCHS) showed that teen sexual activity declined or leveled off in the 1990s through the mid-2000s, and that contraceptive use increased or stabilized.

Chapter 46

Abstinence Versus Comprehensive Sexuality Education

National Data Shows Comprehensive Sex Education Better At Reducing Teen Pregnancy Than Abstinence-Only Programs

Description

Researchers at the University of Washington set out to compare the sexual health risk of adolescents who have received various types of sexuality education. Though a number of recent studies have evaluated specific programs, little research has been done on the adolescent population as a whole.

This study used data collected in 2002–03 through the National Survey of Family Growth (NSFG), a nationwide survey conducted by the Centers for Disease Control and Prevention's (CDC) National Center for Health Statistics.

The researchers analyzed data from 1,719 heterosexual respondents to the NSFG who were 15–19.[1] The median age of respondents was 17. The authors focused on young people's answers to two questions: whether they had received "any formal instruction at school, church, a community center, or some other place about how to say no to sex" before the age of 18 and whether they had received any formal education about birth control. Young people who reported only receiving information on how to say no to sex were classified as participants in abstinence-only programs and young people who reported getting both messages were classified as having received comprehensive sex education. These two groups were also compared to young people who reported receiving no formal sex education.

To assess sexual risk researchers looked at whether respondents reported ever having engaged in vaginal intercourse, been involved in a pregnancy, or been diagnosed with a sexually transmitted disease (STD).

Source

Pamela Kohler, et al., "Abstinence-Only and Comprehensive Sex Education and the Initiation of Sexual Activity and Teen Pregnancy," *Journal of Adolescent Health* 42.4 (March 2008); 344–351.

Key Findings

- Young people who received comprehensive sex education were significantly less likely to report a teen pregnancy compared to those who received no sex education.

- Abstinence-only programs were not significantly associated with a risk reduction for teen pregnancy when compared with no sex education.

- In comparing abstinence-only programs with comprehensive sex education, comprehensive sex education was associated with a 50% lower risk of teen pregnancy.

- After adjusting for demographics, abstinence-only programs were not significantly associated with a delay in the initiation of vaginal intercourse.

- Comprehensive sex education was marginally associated with reduced reports of vaginal intercourse.

- Neither abstinence-only programs nor comprehensive sex education were significantly associated with risk for an STD when compared to no sex education.

Demographic Findings

- Young people who received no sex education tended to be black, from low-income non-intact[2] families, and rural areas.

- Young people who received abstinence-only programs tended to be younger and from low-to-moderate-income intact families.

- Young people who received comprehensive sex education tended to be slightly older, white, and from higher-income families in more urban areas.

- The strongest predictor for an STD diagnosis was a non-intact family. Adolescents in these families were four times more likely to report having been diagnosed with an STD.

SIECUS Analysis

This study adds to the growing body of research in support of a comprehensive approach to sexuality education. First, it confirms that abstinence-only-until-marriage programs are not effective in changing young people's sexual behavior or preventing negative outcomes such as teen pregnancy. More importantly, however, it confirms that programs that teach young people about both abstinence and contraception/disease prevention are, in fact, effective.

In particular, the authors found that receiving information about birth control in formal sex education was associated with a 50% lower risk of teen pregnancy when compared to receiving information only on abstinence. It also confirmed that talking to young people about birth control does not lead to increased sexual activity or higher STD rates as many critics of comprehensive sexuality education continue to claim.

This study is a welcome addition to the research on sexuality education and youth sexual behavior; however, there are some limitations to the data. The NSFG does not ask detailed questions about sex education. Instead, researchers categorized respondents by their answer to two basic questions. By this narrow definition they found that 66.8% of respondents reported receiving comprehensive sex education, 23.8% reported abstinence-only, and 9.4% reported no sex education. However, no information was available about the quality, context, or duration of either the abstinence-only or comprehensive sex education programs.

SIECUS (the Sexuality Information and Education Council of the United States) defines comprehensive sexuality education as programs that start in kindergarten and continue through 12th grade. These programs include age-appropriate, medically accurate information on a broad set of topics related to sexuality, including human development, relationships, decision-making, abstinence, contraception, and disease prevention. They provide students with opportunities for developing skills as well as learning information.

There is a good chance that many of the students grouped as having received comprehensive sex education did not receive such a thorough program. In fact, very few students do. However, it's encouraging that even programs that simply cover birth control and abstinence can reduce young people's risk of teen pregnancy. And, though we know little about the abstinence-only programs that these students were exposed to, we do know that they withheld information about contraception and we know that this approach has failed to reduce sexual activity, teen pregnancy, or STDs.

In addition, this study also reveals some disturbing disparities in what young people are learning. For example, it found that a plurality, 36.9%, of young people who received no sex education live in households that made less than $20,000. Moreover, the authors note that "generally individuals receiving no sex education tended to be from low-income, nonintact families, black, and from rural areas."

♣ It's A Fact!!

The stated goals of federally funded abstinence-only-until-marriage programs are to delay sexual activity and prevent teen pregnancy and, yet, this research shows again that programs that discuss birth control as well as abstinence do a better job at both of these tasks. This research should encourage policymakers to end funding for failed abstinence-only-until-marriage programs and begin funding programs that work.

❖ **It's A Fact!!**

We know that young people of color and young people from low-income communities are disproportionately affected by teen pregnancy and sexually transmitted diseases. In order to overcome these health disparities, we must ensure that these young people, in particular, receive high quality sexuality education.

References

1. Respondents who reported a sexual orientation other than heterosexual were excluded from the analysis because the programs do not address same-sex behavior.

2. "Intact families" were defined as those where the children resided with the same two biological or adoptive parents since birth.

New Abstinence Program Shows Some Results, Shortcomings

Source

John B. Jemmott III, PhD; Loretta S. Jemmott, PhD, RN; Geoffrey T. Fong, PhD, "Efficacy of a Theory-Based Abstinence-Only Intervention Over 24 Months: A Randomized Controlled Trial With Young Adolescents," *Archives of Pediatric and Adolescent Medicine* (February 2010): 152–159.

Description

This study sought to evaluate the effectiveness of an abstinence-only intervention in delaying sex among young adolescents. In the study, 662 African-American students in grades six and seven were recruited from four public middle schools serving low-income communities in Philadelphia; a population at high risk for unintended pregnancy and sexually transmitted diseases (STDs), including human immunodeficiency virus (HIV). The participating students, who were an average of 12 years old, were randomly assigned to five theory-based programs. The programs consisted of two or three four-hour sessions, and were taught in groups of six to eight students. The sessions were implemented on Saturdays in classrooms at the participating schools.

The programs included an eight-hour abstinence-only intervention, an eight-hour safer sex-only intervention, an eight-hour comprehensive (abstinence and safer sex) intervention, a 12-hour comprehensive intervention, or an eight-hour general health-promotion intervention. The general health-promotion intervention served as the control group for the study. The effectiveness of each program was measured over a period of 24 months with follow-up questions to the participants.

The abstinence-only program presented in this study was not designed to meet the restrictive criteria (known as the A–H definition) that was required in order for programs to qualify for federal abstinence-only-until-marriage funding. For example, Federal Requirement 'B' instructed programs to teach "that abstinence from sexual activity outside marriage is the expected standard for all school age children."[1] In contrast, the abstinence-only intervention presented in this study recommends that students abstain from intercourse "until a time later in life when the adolescent is more prepared to handle the consequences of sex." In addition, program facilitators were explicitly instructed not to criticize the benefits of condom use or allow the view that condoms are ineffective to go uncorrected.

Key Findings

- 23.4% of the sixth and seventh grade student participants reported having had sex prior to the interventions.

- Of students who reported not having had sex before the programs started, the following percentages reported sex during the 24 month follow-up period:

  - 32.6% of the abstinence-only program participants

  - 41.2% of the eight-hour comprehensive program participants

  - 42.4% of the 12-hour comprehensive program participants

  - 46.6% of the health-promotion control group participants

  - 51.8% of the safer sex-only program participants

- The abstinence-only program showed significant delay of sexual initiation among participants in the program.

- The abstinence-only program showed no effect on condom use among participants.

- Both the eight-hour and 12-hour comprehensive programs examined in the study reduced the likelihood of participants having multiple partners in the previous three months.

SIECUS Analysis

This study adds some important new data to the conversation about what type of sexuality education delays sex among young teens, however, it in no way validates previously discredited abstinence-only-until-marriage programs.

The abstinence intervention provided as part of this study clearly represented an exceptional approach to education for adolescents. The level of engagement and involvement with participants, small facilitator-to-student ratio, consistent follow up, and one-on-one sessions were undoubtedly hugely beneficial to participants. SIECUS believes we should certainly strive toward this dedication to the sexual health of our youth, but recognizes that such programs and large investments of resources remain rare and are certainly not the norm in abstinence-only programming. Moreover, we do not feel that this study alone merits a new investment in abstinence-only programming.

❖ It's A Fact!!

The abstinence-only program developed by the Jemmotts for this study did not require abstinence until marriage, did not use fear- and shame-based messages about sex, and refused to let suggestions that condoms are ineffective go unchallenged. These criteria alone would make this program ineligible for the federal funding for abstinence-only programs that has existed for the past 14 years. Therefore, this study leaves intact the significant body of evidence showing that abstinence-only-until-marriage programming is ineffective.

While SIECUS and other leading organizations have always stressed an abstinence-focused approach for young teens and pre-teens, the early age that participants in this study began to have sex underscores the need to introduce protective methods to young people early; before their sexual debut. To implement abstinence-only programming with 12-year-old students, of which nearly 25% have already engaged in sexual intercourse, is highly problematic. As the Society for Adolescent Medicine has pointed out, it is unethical for healthcare providers or health educators to withhold information that young people need to protect themselves and it seems obvious that this group of young people needed information about contraception and condoms.[2]

Instead of abstinence-only interventions, we would rather see the sort of exceptional resources invested in this program devoted to sex education that is ethically sound and strives to create sexually healthy adults, not just temporarily abstinent ones. To do that we need a vast range of programs for different cultures, communities, and age groups that provide young people with the skills to make safe and healthy decisions not only about sexual intercourse and contraceptive use, but about communication, relationships, diversity, and countless other issues that are related to sexuality.

1.   For more information about the A–H definition, see the SIECUS Community Action Kit at the following link: <www.communityactionkit.org/index.cfm?pageId=893>.

2.   John Santelli, "Abstinence-only policies and programs: A position paper of the Society for Adolescent Medicine," *Journal of Adolescent Health* (January 2006): 83–87.

Chapter 47

Birth Control: An Overview

What is contraception?

Contraception (also known as birth control) refers to the many different methods of preventing pregnancy. Abstinence from sexual activity until marriage is the only 100 percent sure contraception. Also, abstinent teens are not at risk for pregnancy or sexually transmitted diseases (STDs), including human immunodeficiency virus (HIV)/acquired immune deficiency syndrome (AIDS). Teens who choose to be sexually active should remain faithful (not have sex with anyone else) to reduce the possibility of getting or giving someone a STD or HIV/AIDS. The latex condom is the only contraceptive method that may provide protection against some STDs, including HIV/AIDS. Research shows that latex condoms may not be effective against some STDs such as Human Papilloma Virus (HPV—the virus that causes genital warts).

Who needs contraception?

Anyone who has sex and doesn't want to get pregnant or get someone pregnant needs contraception. Any time you have sex there is a risk of pregnancy. Not having sex—abstinence—is the only 100 percent sure way to avoid pregnancy.

About This Chapter: Information in this chapter is from "What You Should Know About Contraception!" a publication of the U.S. Department of Health and Human Services, March 2003. Reviewed by David A. Cooke, MD, FACP, October 2010.

Are some methods of contraception better than others at preventing pregnancy?

Yes. Abstinence is the only 100 percent sure way to not get pregnant. If you choose to have sex, know that some contraception methods are more effective than others, but no other method offers you total assurance. To be effective, whatever method you choose must be used correctly and consistently. Always read and follow the package instructions. It is a good idea to discuss this with your health care provider.

Is the condom the only kind of contraception for males?

❖ **It's A Fact!!**
Four out of five teens under age 16 have never had sex.

No. Vasectomy is a permanent method of contraception. But the condom is the most common method used by young males. Remember, the condom not only protects you from getting (or getting someone) pregnant, it may also provide protection against HIV/AIDS and some other STDs.

How do I decide which method of contraception to use?

Your health care provider can help you decide which method is best for you. Remember, even if you are using a method like the pill, the latex condom is the only method that may provide some protection against HIV/AIDS and some STDs.

Do I need a prescription to get contraception?

Latex condoms can be purchased without a prescription, but other methods require one. Even if you use a nonprescription method, it is a good idea to see a health care provider on a regular basis.

❖ It's A Fact!!

Contraception is both partners' responsibility. Every baby has a father and a mother, and both males and females can get STDs, including HIV/AIDS.

What are hormonal methods of contraception?

Hormonal methods prevent pregnancy by interrupting the normal process for becoming pregnant. Hormonal methods do not protect against STDs. Hormonal methods include:

- **Emergency Contraception:** Hormonal pills that are taken within 72 hours of unprotected sex or method failure (e.g., the condom broke or you forgot to take your pill). Emergency contraception is the only method that can be used after having sex to prevent pregnancy.

- **Hormonal Implant:** Small capsules inserted under the skin of a woman's upper arm that release small amounts of a hormone.

- **Hormonal Injection:** A hormone injection ("shot") that is injected into a woman's arm or buttock on a regular basis (every one to three months, depending on the hormones).

- **Hormonal Patch:** A thin beige patch containing hormones that a woman applies to her skin once a week for three weeks. Hormones that prevent pregnancy are released during the time the patch is on. The woman removes it for one week, during which time she has her period.

- **The Pill:** A pill that a woman must take at the same time every day.

- **Vaginal Ring:** A ring containing hormones that a woman puts into her vagina and leaves there for three weeks. Hormones that prevent pregnancy are released for that time. The woman removes it for one week, during which time she has her period.

> **❖ It's A Fact!!**
> 82% of all teen pregnancies are unintended.

What are barrier methods of contraception?

Barrier methods prevent sperm from reaching the egg. Barrier methods include:

- **Condom/Rubber:** A cover for the penis or vagina. Latex condoms may provide protection against some STDs, including HIV/AIDS.

❖ It's A Fact!!

A girl can get pregnant if it's her first time having sex. If she has sex, she can become pregnant even if she has never had a period. It is important to know that the menstrual cycle begins before the menstrual period. Girls can ovulate (release an egg) and become pregnant before seeing their first period.

- **Diaphragm/Cervical Cap:** A shallow latex cup which the woman puts into her vagina, covering the cervix, before having sex. The diaphragm is generally used with a spermicidal jelly or cream that stops or kills sperm.

What are other methods of contraception?

- **Abstinence**: Not having vaginal, oral, or anal intercourse. Abstinence is the only 100 percent effective way to prevent pregnancy and STDs, including HIV/AIDS.

- **Intra-Uterine Device (IUD):** An IUD is a small plastic device that is inserted into a woman's uterus by a trained clinician. Those used in the U.S. contain copper or hormones. This method is not generally recommended for teens, but is excellent for faithful married couples.

- **Natural Family Planning:** Not having sex during the five or six days of the month when it is possible for the woman to get pregnant. Specialized training is essential for using this method.

- **Spermicide:** A cream, foam, jelly, or insert which kills sperm. Spermicides do not protect against STDs or HIV/AIDS. Nonoxynol-9, the most common spermicide, may increase the risk of HIV/AIDS in individuals who are at risk for an STD or HIV/AIDS.

- **Sterilization:** A permanent, surgical form of contraception that blocks the fallopian tubes in women (tubal ligation) and the vas deferens in men (vasectomy).

- **Withdrawal:** Removing the penis from the vagina before ejaculation. It may not prevent pregnancy, because some semen may leak before ejaculation.

Chapter 48

Barrier Birth Control Methods

Male Condom (Latex Or Polyurethane)

The male condom is a thin film sheath placed over the erect penis to stop sperm from reaching the egg. Follow these instructions to use a male condom:

• Put it on the erect penis right before sex.

• Pull out before the penis softens.

• Hold the condom against the base of the penis before you pull out.

• Use it only once and then throw it away.

You do not need a prescription for a male condom; you can buy it over the counter.

The risks of the condom are irritation and allergic reactions. If you are allergic to latex, you can try condoms made of polyurethane.

Female Condom

The female condom is a lubricated, thin polyurethane pouch that is put into the vagina. Follow these instructions to use a female condom:

About This Chapter: Information in this chapter is from "Birth Control Guide," a publication of the Food and Drug Administration's Office of Women's Health, April 2010.

- Put the female condom into the vagina right before sex.

- Use it only once and then throw it away.

- You need a new female condom each time you have sex.

You do not need a prescription; you can buy it over the counter. The risks of the female condom are irritation and allergic reactions.

> ♣ **It's A Fact!!**
>
> Except for abstinence, latex condoms are the best protection against human immunodeficiency virus (HIV) and acquired immune deficiency syndrome (AIDS) and other sexually transmitted diseases (STDs). Condoms are the only contraceptive product that may protect against most STDs.

Diaphragm With Spermicide

A diaphragm, a dome-shaped flexible disk with a flexible rim, is made from latex rubber or silicone. It covers the cervix so that sperm cannot reach the egg. Follow these instructions to use a diaphragm:

- You need to put spermicidal jelly on the inside of the diaphragm before putting it into the vagina.

- You must put the diaphragm into the vagina before having sex.

- You must leave the diaphragm in place at least six hours after having sex.

- It can be left in place for up to 24 hours. You need to use more spermicide every time you have sex.

You need a prescription for a diaphragm, and a doctor or nurse will need to do an exam to find the right size diaphragm for you. You should have the diaphragm checked after childbirth or if you lose more than 15 pounds because you might need a different size.

> ♣ **It's A Fact!!**
> The female condom may give some protection against STDs, but it is not as effective as latex condoms. More research is needed.

♣ **It's A Fact!!**

The following birth control methods do **NOT** protect you from STDs: diaphragms, sponges, cervical caps, and spermicides.

The risks of using a diaphragm are:

• You could develop irritation, allergic reactions, and/or a urinary tract infection.

• If you keep it in place longer than 24 hours, there is a risk of toxic shock syndrome. Toxic shock is a rare but serious infection.

Sponge With Spermicide

A sponge is a disk-shaped polyurethane device with the spermicide nonoxynol-9. Follow these instructions to use a sponge:

♣ **It's A Fact!!**

Sponges and cervical caps may not work as well for women who have given birth. Childbirth stretches the vagina and cervix and the sponge or cap may not fit as well.

• Put it into the vagina before you have sex.

• It protects for up to 24 hours. You do not need to use more spermicide each time you have sex.

• You must leave the sponge in place for at least six hours after having sex.

• You must take the sponge out within 30 hours after you put it in. Throw it away after you use it.

You do not need a prescription for the sponge; you can buy it over the counter. The risks of using the sponge are:

• You could develop irritation and allergic reactions.

• Some women may have a hard time taking the sponge out.

• If you keep it in place longer than 24–30 hours, there is a risk of toxic shock syndrome. Toxic shock is a rare but serious infection.

Cervical Cap With Spermicide

A cervical cap is a soft latex or silicone cup with a round rim which fits snugly around the cervix. It covers the cervix so that sperm cannot reach the egg. Follow these instructions to use a cervical cap:

Table 48.1 How effective are barrier methods of birth control?

Out of 100 women who use this method for one year	This number may get pregnant
Male condom*	11–16
Female condom	20
Diaphragm with spermicide	15
Sponge with spermicide	16–32
Cervical cap with spermicide	17–23
Spermicide alone**	About 30

*It is very important to use a male condom each time you have sex.

**Different studies show different rates of effectiveness for spermicide alone.

- Put spermicidal jelly inside the cap before you use it.

- Put the cap in the vagina before you have sex.

- You may find it hard to put in.

- Leave the cap in place for at least six hours after having sex.

- You may leave the cap in for up to 48 hours.

- You do **NOT** need to use more spermicide each time you have sex.

  You need a prescription for the cap. The risks of using the cap are:

- You could develop irritation and/or allergic reactions. You could also have an abnormal Pap test.

- If you keep it in place longer than 48 hours, there is a risk of toxic shock syndrome. Toxic shock is a rare but serious infection.

Spermicide Alone

Spermicide is a foam, cream, jelly, film, or tablet that kills sperm. When using spermicide, keep the following points in mind:

- Instructions can be different for each type of spermicide. Read the label before you use it.

- You need to put spermicide into the vagina between five and 90 minutes before you have sex.

- You usually need to leave it in place at least six to eight hours after; do not douche or rinse the vagina for at least six hours after sex.

You do not need a prescription; you can buy it over the counter. The risks of using spermicide are:

- You could develop irritation, allergic reactions, and/or a urinary tract infection.

- If you are also using a medicine for a vaginal yeast infection, the spermicide might not work as well.

Chapter 49

Using Condoms (Male And Female)

Male Condoms

Consistent and correct use of the male latex condom reduces the risk of sexually transmitted disease (STD) and human immunodeficiency virus (HIV) transmission. However, condom use cannot provide absolute protection against any STD. The most reliable ways to avoid transmission of STDs are to abstain from sexual activity or to be in a long-term mutually monogamous relationship with an uninfected partner. However, many infected persons may be unaware of their infection because STDs often are asymptomatic and unrecognized.

Condom effectiveness for STD and HIV prevention has been demonstrated by both laboratory and epidemiologic studies. Evidence of condom effectiveness is also based on theoretical and empirical data regarding the transmission of different STDs, the physical properties of condoms, and the anatomic coverage or protection provided by condoms.

Epidemiologic studies that compare rates of HIV infection between condom users and nonusers who have HIV-infected sex partners demonstrate that consistent condom use is highly effective in preventing transmission of HIV.

About This Chapter: This chapter begins with "Male Condoms," from "Condom Fact Sheet In Brief," a publication of the Centers for Disease Control and Prevention, April 2010. It concludes with "Instructions for female condoms, © 2005 American Social Health Association (www.ashastd.org). Reprinted with permission. Reviewed by David A. Cooke, MD, FACP, October 2010.

❖ It's A Fact!!

Laboratory studies have shown that latex condoms provide an effective barrier against even the smallest STD pathogens.

Source: Centers for Disease Control and Prevention, April 2010.

Similarly, epidemiologic studies have shown that condom use reduces the risk of many other STDs. However, the exact magnitude of protection has been difficult to quantify because of numerous methodological challenges inherent in studying private behaviors that cannot be directly observed or measured.

Condoms can be expected to provide different levels of protection for various STDs, depending on differences in how the diseases or infections are transmitted. Male condoms may not cover all infected areas or areas that could become infected. Thus, they are likely to provide greater protection against STDs that are transmitted only by genital fluids (STDs such as gonorrhea, chlamydia, trichomoniasis, and HIV infection) than against infections that are transmitted primarily by skin-to-skin contact, which may or may not infect areas covered by a condom (STDs such as genital herpes, human papillomavirus [HPV] infection, syphilis, and chancroid).

How To Use A Condom Consistently And Correctly

- Use a new condom for every act of vaginal, anal, and oral sex throughout the entire sex act (from start to finish).

- Before any genital contact, put the condom on the tip of the erect penis with the rolled side out.

- If the condom does not have a reservoir tip, pinch the tip enough to leave a half-inch space for semen to collect. Holding the tip, unroll the condom all the way to the base of the erect penis.

- After ejaculation and before the penis gets soft, grip the rim of the condom and carefully withdraw. Then gently pull the condom off the penis, making sure that semen doesn't spill out.

- Wrap the condom in a tissue and throw it in the trash where others won't handle it.

- If you feel the condom break at any point during sexual activity, stop immediately, withdraw, remove the broken condom, and put on a new condom.

- Ensure that adequate lubrication is used during vaginal and anal sex, which might require water-based lubricants. Oil-based lubricants (e.g., petroleum jelly, shortening, mineral oil, massage oils, body lotions, and cooking oil) should not be used because they can weaken latex, causing breakage.

❖ It's A Fact!!
Consistent And Correct Condom Use

You must use condoms consistently and correctly to achieve maximum protection. The failure of condoms to protect against STD/HIV transmission usually results from inconsistent or incorrect use, rather than product failure.

Consistent and correct use of latex condoms:

- is highly effective in preventing sexual transmission of HIV, the virus that causes acquired immune deficiency syndrome (AIDS);

- reduces the risk for many STDs that are transmitted by genital fluids;

- reduces the risk for genital ulcer diseases, such as genital herpes, syphilis, and chancroid, only when the infected area or site of potential exposure is protected; and

- may reduce the risk for HPV infection and HPV-associated diseases (e.g., genital warts and cervical cancer).

Source: Centers for Disease Control and Prevention, April 2010.

✤ It's A Fact!!

• Inconsistent condom use or nonuse can lead to STD acquisition because transmission can occur with a single sex act with an infected partner.

• Incorrect condom use diminishes the protective effect of condoms by leading to condom breakage, slippage, or leakage. Incorrect use more commonly entails a failure to use condoms throughout the entire sex act, from start (of sexual contact) to finish (after ejaculation).

Source: Centers for Disease Control and Prevention, April 2010.

Instructions For Female Condoms

The female condom is a polyurethane (plastic) pouch that fits inside a woman's vagina. It has a soft ring on each end. The outer ring stays on the outside of the vagina and partly covers the labia (lips). The inner ring fits on the inside of the vagina, somewhat like a diaphragm, to hold the condom in place.

Insert the condom any time before the penis touches the vagina. Add lubricant to the inside of the condom. Squeeze the inner ring of the condom. Put the inner ring and pouch inside the vagina.

With your finger, push the inner ring as far into the vagina as it will go. The outer ring stays outside the vagina. Guide the penis into the condom. Remove the condom before standing up. Pull out gently.

Chapter 50

Other Birth Control Methods

Hormonal Methods

Oral Contraceptives ("The Pill"): Combined Pill

The combined pill uses hormones (estrogen and progestin) to stop the ovaries from releasing eggs in most women. It also thickens the cervical mucus, which keeps the sperm from joining with the egg.

Risks for the combined pill include:

• dizziness

• nausea

• changes in your cycle (period)

• changes in mood

• weight gain

Oral Contraceptives ("The Pill"): Progestin-Only

The progestin-only pill only has the hormone progestin. It thickens the cervical mucus, which keeps sperm from joining with an egg. Less often, it stops the ovaries from releasing eggs.

About This Chapter: Information in this chapter is from "Birth Control Guide," a publication of the Food and Drug Administration's Office of Women's Health, April 2010.

The risks of taking this pill are:

- irregular bleeding

- weight gain

- breast tenderness

- less protection against ectopic pregnancy (pregnancy in the fallopian tubes) than the combination pill

<table>
<tr><td>

✤ It's A Fact!!

- It is not common, but some women who take the pill develop high blood pressure.

- It is rare, but some women will have blood clots, heart attacks, or strokes.

</td></tr>
</table>

Oral Contraceptives ("The Pill"): Extended/Continuous Use

The extended/continuous use pill uses hormones (estrogen and progestin) to stop the ovaries from releasing eggs in most women. It also thickens the cervical mucus, which keeps the sperm from joining with the egg. These pills are designed so women have fewer or no periods.

The risks for this kind of pill are similar to other oral contraceptives. In addition:

- You may have fewer planned periods. If you miss a scheduled period, you may be pregnant.

✤ It's A Fact!!
Facts About Oral Contraceptives

Regardless of which type of pill you take, remember:

- You need a prescription to get it.

- You should swallow the pill at the same time every day, whether or not you have sex.

- Out of 100 women who use this method for one year, about five may get pregnant.

- The pill does not protect you from sexually transmitted infections (STIs).

♣ **It's A Fact!!**

The patch may be less effective for women who weigh
more than 198 lbs.

- You will likely have more bleeding and spotting between periods than
  with other oral contraceptives.

Patch

The patch is a skin patch you can wear on the lower abdomen, buttocks,
or upper body. It uses hormones (estrogen and progestin) to stop the ovaries
from releasing eggs in most women. It also thickens the cervical mucus, which
keeps the sperm from joining with the egg.

To use the patch, you put on a new patch and take off the old patch once
a week for three weeks. During the fourth week, you do not wear a patch and
you have a menstrual period.

You need a prescription to get the patch. Out of 100 women who use this
method for one year, about five may get pregnant.

The patch will expose you to higher than average levels of estrogen than
most oral contraceptives. It is not known if serious risks, such as blood clots,
are greater with the skin patch because of the greater exposure to estrogen.

Vaginal Contraceptive Ring

The vaginal contraceptive ring is a two-inch, flexible ring that a woman
puts into her vagina. It releases hormones (progestin and estrogen) to stop
the ovaries from releasing eggs in most women. It also thickens the cervical
mucus, which keeps the sperm from joining with the egg.

When using the ring:

- Put the ring into the vagina yourself.

- Keep the ring in your vagina for three weeks then take it out for one
  week.

- If the ring falls out and stays out for more than three hours, you need to use another kind of birth control method until the ring has been used for seven days in a row.

You need a prescription for the ring. Out of 100 women who use this method for one year, about five may get pregnant.

The risks of using the ring are similar to those for the combined pill. In addition, you might have vaginal discharge, vaginal swelling, and irritation.

Shot/Injection

The shot is a shot of the hormone progestin that stops the ovaries from releasing eggs in most women. It also thickens the cervical mucus, which keeps the sperm from joining with the egg.

You need a prescription for the shot, and you must have one shot every three months. Out of 100 women who use this method for one year, less than one may get pregnant.

The risks of using the shot are:

- possible bone loss if you get the shot for more than two years
- bleeding between periods
- weight gain
- breast tenderness
- headaches

Emergency Contraceptives (The Morning After Pill)

The morning after pill consists of one or two pills with hormones that are similar to other birth control pills. It works by stopping the ovaries from releasing an egg or stopping sperm from joining with the egg.

Be sure to follow the directions when taking the morning after pill:

✤ It's A Fact!!

The hormonal methods of birth control—the pill (including the "morning after" pill), the patch, the ring, and the shot—do **NOT** protect you from sexually transmitted diseases (STDs).

- You can use it after you have unprotected sex (did not use birth control).

- You can also use it if your birth control did not work (for example, the condom broke).

- You must swallow the pill(s) within 72 hours of having unprotected sex.

- For the best chance to prevent a pregnancy, you should start taking the pill(s) as soon as possible after unprotected sex.

❖ **It's A Fact!!**

The morning after pill reduces the risk of pregnancy resulting from a single act of unprotected sex by almost 85 percent, if you take it within 72 hours.

You can buy the morning after pill over the counter if you are 17 years or older. If you are younger than 17, you need a prescription.

Some common side effects are a heavier menstrual period for the next month, nausea, abdominal pain, fatigue, headache, and dizziness.

Implanted Birth Control Methods

Intrauterine Device (IUD)

An IUD is a prescription-only, T-shaped device that is put into the uterus by a healthcare provider. It can stay in place for five to 10 years, depending on the type.

Out of 100 women who use this method for one year, less than one may get pregnant.

The risks of using an IUD are: cramps, bleeding, pelvic inflammatory disease, infertility, and a tear or hole in the uterus.

Implantable Rod

An implantable rod is a thin, matchstick-sized rod that contains the hormone progestin. It thickens the cervical mucus, which keeps sperm from joining with the egg. Less often, it stops the ovaries from releasing eggs.

A doctor or nurse puts the rod under the skin on the inside of your upper arm. You will get a shot in the upper arm to make the skin numb, then the rod is placed just under the skin with a needle. It lasts up to three years.

Out of 100 women who use this method for one year, less than one may get pregnant. However, it might not work as well for overweight or obese women or if you are taking certain medicines for things like tuberculosis (TB), seizures, depression, or human immunodeficiency virus (HIV)/acquired immune deficiency syndrome (AIDS). Tell your doctor if you are taking the herb St. John's wort.

The risks of using the rod are: acne; weight gain; ovarian cysts; mood changes; depression; hair loss; headache; upset stomach; dizziness; lower interest in sexual activity; sore breasts; and changes in your periods.

Sterilization

Sterilization Surgery For Women: Trans-Abdominal Implant

During surgical sterilization, a device is placed on the outside of each fallopian tube. The woman's fallopian tubes are blocked so the egg and sperm can't meet in the fallopian tube. This stops you from getting pregnant.

This is an elective surgery (a surgery you must request) that a woman has only once, and it is permanent. You will need a small incision (cut) below the belly button and two or more smaller incisions.

> ✣ **It's A Fact!!**
> Implanted methods of birth control do **NOT** protect you from sexually transmitted diseases (STDs).

Out of 100 women who use this method for one year, less than one may get pregnant. The risks of this surgery are:

• pain

• bleeding

• infection or other complications after surgery

• ectopic (tubal) pregnancy

Sterilization Surgery For Women: Trans-Cervical Implant

During this surgery, a small flexible metal coil is put into the fallopian tubes through the vagina. The device works by causing scar tissue to form around the coil. This blocks the fallopian tubes and stops you from getting pregnant.

The healthcare provider uses a camera to find the fallopian tubes. Once they are found, the sterilization device is put inside the fallopian tube with a special catheter. No incision is needed; however, you may need local anesthesia. The surgery is permanent.

Out of 100 women who use this method for one year, less than one may get pregnant. The risks of this surgery are mild to moderate pain after insertion and ectopic (tubal) pregnancy.

Sterilization Surgery For Men: Vasectomy

This surgery blocks a man's vas deferens (the tubes that carry sperm from the testes to other glands). Semen (the fluid that comes out of a man's penis) never has any sperm in it. A man has this surgery only once; it is permanent.

Out of 100 women whose partner uses this method for one year, less than one may get pregnant. The risks of the surgery are pain, bleeding, and infection.

Chapter 51

Fertility Awareness

What Is It?

Fertility awareness is a way to prevent pregnancy by not having sex around the time of ovulation (the release of an egg during a girl's monthly cycle). Couples who do want to have a baby can also use this method to have sex during the time that they are most likely to conceive. Fertility awareness can include methods such as natural family planning, periodic abstinence, and the rhythm method.

How Does It Work?

If a couple doesn't have sex around the time of ovulation, the girl is less likely to get pregnant. The trick is knowing when ovulation happens. Couples use a calendar, a thermometer to measure body temperature, the thickness of cervical mucus, or a kit that tests for ovulation. The ovulation kits are more useful for couples who are trying to get pregnant. The fertile period around ovulation lasts six to nine days and during this time the couple using only fertility awareness for birth control who does not want to get pregnant should not have sex.

"Fertility Awareness," April 2010, reprinted with permission from www.kidshealth.org. Copyright © 2010 The Nemours Foundation. This information was provided by Kids Health, one of the largest resources online for medically reviewed health information written for parents, kids, and teens. For more articles like this one, visit www.KidsHealth .org, or www.TeensHealth.org.

How Well Does It Work?

Fertility awareness is not a reliable way to prevent pregnancy for most teens. Over the course of one year, as many as 25 out of 100 typical couples who rely on fertility awareness to prevent pregnancy will have an accidental pregnancy. Of course, this is an average figure, and the chance of getting pregnant depends on whether a couple uses one or more of the fertility awareness methods correctly and consistently and does not have unprotected sex during the fertile period.

In general, how well each type of birth control method works depends on a lot of things. These include whether a person has any health conditions, is taking any medications that might interfere with its use, whether the method chosen is convenient—and whether it is used correctly all the time. In the case of fertility awareness, it also depends on how consistent a woman's ovulatory cycle is, how accurately a couple keeps track of when she could be ovulating, and how reliably unprotected sex is avoided during the fertile period.

Protection Against STDs

Fertility awareness does not protect against sexually transmitted diseases (STDs). Couples having sex must always use condoms along with their chosen method of birth control to protect against STDs.

> ✤ **It's A Fact!!**
> Abstinence (not having sex) is the only method that always prevents pregnancy and STDs.

Who Uses It?

It is often very difficult to tell when a girl is fertile. Because teens often have irregular menstrual cycles, it makes predicting ovulation much more difficult. Even people who have previously had regular cycles can have irregular timing of ovulation when factors such as stress or illness are involved. Fertility awareness also requires a commitment to monitoring body changes, keeping daily records, and above all not having sex during the fertile period.

How Do You Get It?

For couples interested in this method, it is best to talk to a doctor or counselor who is trained in fertility awareness. He or she can then teach the couple the skills they need to know to practice this birth control method accurately.

❖ **It's A Fact!!**
Fertility awareness is not a reliable way to
prevent pregnancy for most teens.

How Much Does It Cost?

The tools needed for fertility awareness—such as ovulation detection kits and thermometers, for example—are available in drugstores. But they can be expensive. Again, it's best to talk to a doctor for advice on using this method.

Chapter 52

Withdrawal

What's with withdrawal?

Pulling out, or the pull-out method, refers to withdrawal, which is one of many ways to prevent pregnancy. Read on for the scoop on withdrawal: how it works, how well it works, and why it may not be the right choice for teens.

What is withdrawal?

Also known—more scientifically—as coitus interruptus, withdrawal may be the world's oldest way to practice birth control. When a guy performs withdrawal, he removes his penis from the vagina before he ejaculates, or comes—that's when semen spurts from his penis.

How does that prevent pregnancy?

The idea behind withdrawal is simple: If sperm is not released into the vagina, pregnancy is impossible.

Does it really work?

Well, that's the thing. In a perfect world, yes, if a guy pulls out in time, pregnancy should be prevented. But there are a couple other factors to consider.

About This Chapter: Information in this chapter is from "What's With Withdrawal?" Reprinted with permission from Planned Parenthood® Federation of America, Inc. © 2010 PPFA. All rights reserved.

First of all, a guy practicing withdrawal needs to really know his body, because he must be able to predict the exact moment when he won't be able to stop ejaculation. If he can't do this, then it's very possible that he won't pull out in time, and pregnancy might not be prevented.

Also, it may be possible for a woman to become pregnant even if withdrawal is performed correctly. Pre-ejaculate—or pre-cum—does not contain sperm. But it can pick up sperm from a previous ejaculation as it passes through the urethra before it seeps out of the tip of the penis during sexual excitement, before ejaculation happens. It can pick up enough sperm to cause pregnancy. (All men ooze pre-ejaculate, whether they know it or not.)

> ♣ **It's A Fact!!**
> The numbers don't lie: Of every 100 women whose partners use withdrawal, four will become pregnant each year if they always do it correctly. And of every 100 women whose partners use withdrawal and don't always do it correctly, 27 will become pregnant each year.

Does withdrawal protect me from sexually transmitted infections (STIs)?

Nope. If practiced correctly, withdrawal can only prevent pregnancy, not the spread of infection. Using a latex or female condom will help reduce the risk of contracting an STI.

How do I practice withdrawal?

During sex, a guy withdraws his penis from the vagina when he feels he is going to ejaculate, or cum—or right before that point. There is a very cool medical term for that moment. It's called "ejaculatory inevitability."

When a guy knows he can't keep from coming—when he reaches ejaculatory inevitability—he has to pull out. He comes outside his partner's vagina, and makes sure semen does not spill onto the vulva. If he is going to have sex again, he should make sure to wipe off his penis and urinate first. This will help flush any sperm out of his urethra.

Are there advantages to using this method?

Yes. Couples who practice withdrawal enjoy that it

- can be used when no other method of birth control is available

- has no medical or hormonal side effects, like some other methods of birth control

- requires no prescription from a health care provider

- is completely free

Are there disadvantages?

There are. The biggest one to pay attention to—and it's a pretty big one—is the risk of performing withdrawal incorrectly.

When considering using withdrawal, it's important to remember that it

- requires a lot of self-control, experience, and trust

- is not a good method for a guy who tends to cum too fast

- is not a good method for a guy who can't always tell when he needs to pull out

- is not a good method for a woman who doesn't know her sex partner very well

So what about withdrawal for a teen like me?

Good question! Withdrawal is not a method of birth control usually recommended for teens. That's because of the risk of performing it incorrectly. Even if he tries really hard to do it right, a younger guy is less experienced when it comes to sex, and therefore may not know his body well enough to perform withdrawal effectively.

✔ Quick Tip

Pulling out can also offer extra protection when you're using other forms of birth control, like the pill, cap, condom, diaphragm, or female condom. So don't be afraid to double up for extra protection!

It's pretty easy for a guy to get caught up in the heat of the moment, and end up coming before he's had a chance to pull out. He may have intended to pull out in time, but missed the point where he could stop himself from ejaculating. Younger guys are also more likely to ejaculate prematurely than older men with more experience.

❖ **It's A Fact!!**
A mistake means sperm is released into the vagina, and it only takes one mistake to result in a pregnancy!

Part Six

Sexually Transmitted Diseases

Chapter 53

Sexually Transmitted Diseases (STDs): An Overview

What are sexually transmitted diseases (STDs)?

STDs, also called sexually transmitted infections or STIs, are diseases that you get by having intimate sexual contact, that is having sex (vaginal, oral, or anal intercourse), with someone who already has the disease. Every year, STDs affect more than 13 million people.

What are the different types of STDs?

Researchers have identified more than 20 different kinds of STDs, which can fall into two main groups:

- **STDs Caused By Bacteria:** These diseases can be treated and often cured with antibiotics. Some bacterial STDs include: chlamydia, gonorrhea, trichomoniasis, and syphilis.

- **STDs Caused By Viruses:** These diseases can be controlled, but not cured. If you get a viral STD, you will always have it. Some viral STDs

About This Chapter: Information in this chapter is from "Sexually Transmitted Diseases (STDs)," a publication of the Eunice Kennedy Shriver National Institute of Child Health and Human Development, May 2007. The chapter also includes information from "STDS Today," a publication of the Centers for Disease Control and Prevention National Prevention Information Network, March 2010.

include: human immunodeficiency virus (HIV)/acquired immune deficiency syndrome (AIDS), genital herpes, genital warts, human papilloma virus (HPV), hepatitis B virus (HBV), and cytomegalovirus.

What are the symptoms of STDs?

The symptoms vary among the different types of STDs. Some examples of common symptoms include the following:

- Unusual discharge from the penis or vagina

- Sores or warts on the genital area

- Burning while urinating

- Itching and redness in the genital area

- Anal itching, soreness, or bleeding

> ✔ **Quick Tip**
>
> If you are having any of the symptoms described in this chapter or think you might have an STD, talk to your health care provider.
>
> Source: National Institute of Child Health and Human Development, May 2007.

How can STDs be prevented?

The only way to ensure that you won't get infected is to not have sex. This means avoiding all types of intimate sexual contact.

If you are sexually active, you can reduce your risk of getting STDs by practicing "safe sex." This means following these guidelines:

- Using a condom for vaginal, oral, and anal intercourse—every time

- Knowing your partner and his/her STD status and health

- Having regular medical checkups, especially if you have more than one sexual partner

What are some common STDs and the organisms that cause them?

Many people are aware of the most prominent STD—HIV. However, many other STDs affect millions of men and women each year. Many of these STDs initially cause no symptoms, especially in women. When symptoms develop, they may be confused with those of other diseases that are not transmitted through sexual contact. STDs can still be transmitted from person to person even if the infected people do not show symptoms. Furthermore, health problems caused by STDs tend to be more severe for women than for men.

Below are descriptions of several of the most common STDs, including information about incidence, symptoms (if any), and treatment.

AIDS: People who have AIDS are very susceptible to many life-threatening diseases, called opportunistic infections, and to certain forms of cancer. Transmission of the virus primarily occurs during unprotected sexual activity and by sharing needles used to inject intravenous drugs.

Chancroid: Chancroid is a bacterial infection caused by *Haemophilus ducreyi*, which is spread by sexual contact and results in genital ulcers. The disease is found primarily in developing and Third World countries. People with chancroid can be treated effectively with one of several antibiotics.

Chlamydia: Chlamydial infection is a common STD caused by the bacterium *Chlamydia trachomatis*. Chlamydia is the most frequently reported bacterial STD in the United States. Even though symptoms of chlamydia are usually mild or absent, it can damage a woman's reproductive organs and cause serious complications. Irreversible damage, including infertility, can occur "silently" before a woman ever recognizes a problem. Chlamydia also can cause discharge from the penis of an infected man, although complications among men are rare. Chlamydia can be easily treated and cured with antibiotics.

Genital Herpes/Herpes Simplex Virus (HSV): Genital herpes is a contagious viral infection caused by the herpes simplex virus (HSV). There are two types of HSV: herpes simplex virus type 1 (HSV-1) and type 2 (HSV-2). Both can cause genital herpes, although most genital herpes is caused by HSV-2. Most individuals have no or only minimal signs or symptoms from HSV-1 or HSV-2 infection. There is no treatment that can cure herpes, but antiviral medications can shorten and prevent outbreaks during the period of time the person takes the medication.

Genital HPV Infection: HPV is the most common STD. There are more than 40 HPV types that can infect the genital areas of males and females. These HPV types can also infect the mouth and throat. Low-risk types of HPV cause genital warts, the most recognizable sign of genital HPV infection. Other high-risk types of HPV cause cervical cancer and other genital cancers.

Vaccines can protect males and females against some of the most common types of HPV. These vaccines are given in three shots. It is important to get all three doses to get the best protection. The vaccines are most effective when given before a person's first sexual contact, when he or she could be exposed to HPV.

Gonorrhea: Gonorrhea is caused by *Neisseria gonorrhoeae*, a bacterium that can grow and multiply easily in the warm, moist areas of the reproductive tract. The most common symptoms of infection are a discharge from the vagina or penis and painful or difficult urination. The most common and serious complications occur in women.

> **❖ It's A Fact!!**
> Most people with HPV do not develop symptoms or health problems. In 90 percent of cases, the body's immune system clears the HPV infection naturally within two years.
>
> Source: Centers for Disease Control and Prevention, March 2010.

Several antibiotics can successfully cure gonorrhea in adolescents and adults. However, antibiotic-resistant strains of gonorrhea are increasing in many areas of the world, including the United States, and successful treatment of gonorrhea is becoming more difficult. New antibiotics or combinations of drugs must be used to treat these resistant strains.

Syphilis: Syphilis is caused by the bacterium *Treponema pallidum*. Syphilis is passed from person to person through direct contact with syphilis sores. The first symptoms of syphilis infection may go undetected because they are very mild and disappear spontaneously. The initial symptom is a chancre (genital sore); it is usually a painless open sore that most often appears on the penis or around or in the vagina. It can also occur near the mouth or anus or on the hands.

If untreated, syphilis may go on to more advanced stages, including a transient rash, and eventually can cause serious damage to the brain, nerves, eyes, heart, blood vessels, liver, bones, and joints. The full course of the disease can take years.

Penicillin remains the most effective drug to treat people with syphilis. For people who are allergic to penicillin, other antibiotics are available to treat syphilis.

Trichomoniasis: Trichomoniasis is caused by the single-celled protozoan parasite, *Trichomonas vaginalis*. It is the most common curable STD in young, sexually active women, and it affects men as well although symptoms are most common in women. Trichomoniasis can usually be cured with prescription drugs, either metronidazole or tinidazole, given by mouth in a single dose.

Viral Hepatitis: Hepatitis B is a serious liver infection caused by hepatitis B virus (HBV). HBV infection can cause acute illness and lead to chronic or lifelong infection, cirrhosis (scarring) of the liver, liver cancer, liver failure, and death. HBV is transmitted through percutaneous (puncture through the skin) or mucosal contact with infectious blood or body fluids. Hepatitis B vaccination is the most effective measure to prevent HBV infection and its consequences and is recommended for all infants and others at risk for HBV infection.

Hepatitis C is a liver disease caused by the hepatitis C virus (HCV) that sometimes results in an acute illness, but most often becomes a silent, chronic infection that can lead to cirrhosis (scarring) of the liver, liver failure, liver cancer, and death. Chronic HCV infection develops in a majority of HCV-infected persons, most of whom do not know they are infected since they have no symptoms. There is no vaccine for hepatitis C.

Other STDs: Other diseases that may be sexually transmitted include bacterial vaginosis, scabies, pubic "crab" lice, and pelvic inflammatory disease (PID).

Who is being infected?

In the United States alone, an estimated 19 million new STD infections occur each year. STDs affect men and women of all backgrounds and economic levels. However, there are clear disparities.

Women, especially young and minority women, are hardest hit by chlamydia. In 2008, girls 15 to 19 years of age had the highest numbers of reported cases (342,875) and rates of chlamydia (3,275.8 per 100,000 females), followed closely by young women 20 to 24 years of age (323,696 cases; 3,179.9 cases per 100,000 females).

CDC's 2008 STD surveillance report found persistent racial disparities in STD rates. Blacks represent only 12 percent of the total U.S. population but made up more than 70 percent of gonorrhea cases. The syphilis rate among blacks was about eight times higher than that of whites in 2008, and the chlamydia rate was more than eight times higher than that of whites. Disparities among Hispanics also exist, with chlamydia rates almost three times higher than those of whites, and gonorrhea and syphilis rates double those of whites. Gonorrhea rates among American Indian/Alaska Natives were 3.6 times higher than those of whites, and chlamydia rates were 4.7 times higher.

The majority of reported syphilis cases in the United States continues to be among men who have sex with men (MSM). In 2008, data from the District of Columbia and the 44 states that track the gender of sex partners of those infected with syphilis showed that 63 percent of primary and secondary syphilis cases were among MSM, compared to only four percent of cases in 2000. This is of particular concern, since MSM are also most heavily affected by HIV, and syphilis infection can facilitate HIV transmission.

Chapter 54

STD Prevention

Despite the fact that a great deal of progress has been made in sexually transmitted disease (STD) prevention over the past four decades, the United States has the highest rates of STD infection in the industrialized world, making prevention as important as ever.

Preventing STD Infection

The following are the most reliable ways to avoid becoming infected with or transmitting STDs:

- Abstain from sexual intercourse (i.e., oral, vaginal, or anal sex).

- Be in a long-term, mutually monogamous relationship with an uninfected partner.

- Latex male condoms, when used consistently and correctly, can reduce the risk of transmission of chlamydia, gonorrhea, and trichomoniasis.

Reducing Your Risk Of STD Infection

All partners should get tested for human immunodeficiency virus (HIV) and other STDs before initiating sexual intercourse. However, if you decide

About This Chapter: Information in this chapter is from "STD Prevention Today," a publication of the Centers for Disease Control and Prevention, August 2010; and "Condoms and STDs: Fact Sheet for Public Health Personnel," Centers for Disease Control and Prevention, February 2010.

to be sexually active with a partner whose infection status is unknown or who is infected with HIV or another STD, you can reduce your risk of contracting an STD:

- **Ask a new sex partner if he or she has an STD, has been exposed to one, or has any unexplained physical symptoms.** Do not have unprotected sex if your partner has signs or symptoms of STDs, such as sores, rashes, or discharge from the genital area. Many common STDs have no symptoms but can still be transmitted to a sexual partner. If your partner has had sexual relations with someone else recently, he or she may have an STD, even if there are no symptoms.

- **Use a new condom for each act of insertive intercourse.** Correct and consistent use of latex condoms and other barriers can reduce the risk of transmission only when the infected area or site of potential exposure is protected.

- **Get regular checkups for STDs (even if you show no symptoms), and be familiar with the common symptoms.** Most STDs are readily treated, and the earlier treatment is sought and sex partners are notified, the less likely the disease will do irreparable damage.

✤ It's A Fact!!
Sexually Transmitted Diseases, Including HIV Infection

Latex condoms, when used consistently and correctly, are highly effective in preventing the sexual transmission of HIV, the virus that causes acquired immune deficiency syndrome (AIDS). In addition, consistent and correct use of latex condoms reduces the risk of other STDs, including diseases transmitted by genital secretions, and to a lesser degree, genital ulcer diseases. Condom use may reduce the risk for genital human papillomavirus (HPV) infection and HPV-associated diseases, e.g., genital warts and cervical cancer.

Source: Centers for Disease Control and Prevention, February 2010.

> ### ❖ It's A Fact!!
> Although consistent and correct use of condoms is inherently difficult to measure because such studies would involve observations of private behaviors, several published studies have demonstrated that failure to measure these factors properly tends to result in underestimation of condom effectiveness.
>
> Source: Centers for Disease Control and Prevention, February 2010.

Condoms And STDs

Consistent and correct use of male latex condoms can reduce (though not eliminate) the risk of STD transmission. To achieve the maximum protective effect, condoms must be used both consistently and correctly. Inconsistent use can lead to STD acquisition because transmission can occur with a single act of intercourse with an infected partner. Similarly, if condoms are not used correctly, the protective effect may be diminished even when they are used consistently. The most reliable ways to avoid transmission of sexually transmitted diseases, including HIV, are to abstain from sexual activity or to be in a long-term mutually monogamous relationship with an uninfected partner. However, many infected persons may be unaware of their infections because STDs are often asymptomatic or unrecognized.

There are two primary ways that STDs are transmitted. Some diseases, such as HIV infection, gonorrhea, chlamydia, and trichomoniasis, are transmitted when infected urethral or vaginal secretions contact mucosal surfaces (such as the male urethra, the vagina, or cervix). In contrast, genital ulcer diseases (such as genital herpes, syphilis, and chancroid) and human papillomavirus (HPV) infection are primarily transmitted through contact with infected skin or mucosal surfaces.

Condoms can be expected to provide different levels of protection for various STDs, depending on differences in how the diseases are transmitted. Condoms block transmission and acquisition of STDs by preventing contact between the condom wearer's penis and a sex partner's skin, mucosa, and genital secretions. A greater level of protection is provided for the diseases transmitted by genital secretions. A lesser degree of protection is provided for genital ulcer diseases or HPV because these infections also may be transmitted by exposure to areas (e.g., infected skin or mucosal surfaces) that are not covered or protected by the condom.

HIV, The Virus That Causes AIDS: HIV infection is, by far, the most deadly STD, and considerably more scientific evidence exists regarding condom effectiveness for prevention of HIV infection than for other STDs. The body of research on the effectiveness of latex condoms in preventing sexual transmission of HIV is both comprehensive and conclusive. The ability of latex condoms to prevent transmission of HIV has been scientifically established in "real-life" studies of sexually active couples as well as in laboratory studies. Laboratory studies have demonstrated that latex condoms provide an essentially impermeable barrier to particles the size of HIV.

Other Diseases Transmitted By Genital Secretions: Latex condoms, when used consistently and correctly, reduce the risk of transmission of STDs such as gonorrhea, chlamydia, and trichomoniasis. These diseases are sexually transmitted by genital secretions, such as urethral or vaginal secretions.

Genital Ulcer Diseases And HPV Infections: Genital ulcer diseases include genital herpes, syphilis, and chancroid. These diseases are transmitted primarily through "skin-to-skin" contact from sores/ulcers or infected skin that looks normal. HPV infections are transmitted through contact with infected genital skin or mucosal surfaces/secretions. Genital ulcer diseases and HPV infection can occur in male or female genital areas that are covered (protected by the condom) as well as those areas that are not.

✤ It's A Fact!!

Consistent and correct use of latex condoms reduces the risk of genital herpes, syphilis, and chancroid only when the infected area or site of potential exposure is protected. Condom use may reduce the risk for HPV infection and HPV-associated diseases (e.g., genital warts and cervical cancer).

Source: Centers for Disease Control and Prevention, February 2010.

✔ **Quick Tip**

While condom use has been associated with a lower risk of cervical cancer, the use of condoms should not be a substitute for routine screening with Pap smears to detect and prevent cervical cancer, nor should it be a substitute for HPV vaccination among those eligible for the vaccine.

Source: Centers for Disease Control and Prevention, February 2010.

Epidemiologic studies that compare infection rates among condom users and nonusers provide evidence that latex condoms provide limited protection against syphilis and herpes simplex virus-2 transmission. No conclusive studies have specifically addressed the transmission of chancroid and condom use, although several studies have documented a reduced risk of genital ulcers associated with increased condom use in settings where chancroid is a leading cause of genital ulcers.

Condom use may reduce the risk for HPV-associated diseases (e.g., genital warts and cervical cancer) and may mitigate the other adverse consequences of infection with HPV; condom use has been associated with higher rates of regression of cervical intraepithelial neoplasia (CIN) and clearance of HPV infection in women, and with regression of HPV-associated penile lesions in men. A limited number of prospective studies have demonstrated a protective effect of condoms on the acquisition of genital HPV.

Chapter 55

Chlamydia

What is chlamydia and how common is it?

Chlamydia is a sexually transmitted infection (STI). STIs are also called STDs, or sexually transmitted diseases. Chlamydia is an STI caused by bacteria called *Chlamydia trachomatis*. Chlamydia is the most commonly reported STI in the United States. Women, especially young women, are hit hardest by chlamydia.

Women often get chlamydia more than once, meaning they are reinfected. This can happen if their sex partners were not treated. Reinfections place women at higher risk for serious reproductive health problems, such as infertility.

How do you get chlamydia?

You get chlamydia from vaginal, anal, or oral sex with an infected person. Chlamydia often has no symptoms. So people who are infected may pass chlamydia to their sex partners without knowing it. The more sex partners you (or your partner) have, the higher your risk of getting this STI.

An infected mother can pass chlamydia to her baby during childbirth. Babies born to infected mothers can get pneumonia or infections in their eyes.

About This Chapter: Information in this chapter is from "Chlamydia: Frequently Asked Questions," a publication of the U.S. Department of Health and Human Services, Office on Women's Health, March 2009.

What are the symptoms of chlamydia?

Chlamydia is known as a silent disease. This is because 75 percent of infected women and at least half of infected men have no symptoms. If symptoms do occur, they most often appear within one to three weeks of exposure. The infection first attacks the cervix and urethra. Even if the infection spreads to the uterus and fallopian tubes, some women still have no symptoms. If you do have symptoms, you may have: abnormal vaginal discharge; burning when passing urine; lower abdominal pain; low back pain; nausea; fever; pain during sex; and bleeding between periods.

Men with chlamydia may have: discharge from the penis; burning when passing urine; burning and itching around the opening of the penis; pain and swelling in the testicles.

Chlamydia is often not diagnosed or treated until problems show up. If you think you may have chlamydia, both you and your sex partner(s) should see a doctor right away—even if you have no symptoms.

Chlamydia can be confused with gonorrhea, another STI. These STIs have some of the same symptoms and problems if not treated. But they have different treatments.

How is chlamydia diagnosed?

A doctor can diagnose chlamydia through a swab test, where a fluid sample from an infected site (cervix or penis) is tested for the bacteria or a urine test, where a urine sample is tested for the bacteria.

Who should get tested for chlamydia?

You should be tested for chlamydia once a year if these characteristics describe you:

- 25 or younger and have sex

- Older than 25 and any of the following:

    - Have a new sex partner

    - Have more than one sex partner

✤ **It's A Fact!!**
The chlamydia bacteria also can infect your throat if you have oral sex with an infected partner.

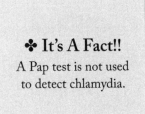

❖ It's A Fact!!
A Pap test is not used to detect chlamydia.

- Have sex with someone who has other sex partners

- Fail to use a condom during sex within a relationship that is not mutually monogamous, meaning you or your partner has sex with other people

- Pregnant

You also should be tested if you have any symptoms of chlamydia.

What is the treatment for chlamydia?

Antibiotics are used to treat chlamydia. If treated, chlamydia can be cured.

All sex partners should be treated to keep from getting chlamydia again. Do not have sex until you and your sex partner(s) have ended treatment.

✔ Quick Tip

Tell your doctor if you are pregnant. Your doctor can give you an antibiotic that is commonly used during pregnancy.

What should I do if I have chlamydia?

Chlamydia is easy to treat. But you should be tested and treated right away to protect your reproductive health. If you have chlamydia, follow these guidelines:

- **See a doctor right away.** Women with chlamydia are five times more likely to get human immunodeficiency virus (HIV), the virus that causes acquired immune deficiency syndrome (AIDS), from an infected partner.

- **Follow your doctor's orders and finish all your antibiotics.** Even if symptoms go away, you need to finish all the medicine.

- **Don't engage in any sexual activity while being treated for chlamydia.**

- **Tell your sex partner(s) so they can be treated.**

- **See your doctor again if your symptoms don't go away within one to two weeks after finishing the medicine.**

- **See your doctor again within three to four months for another chlamydia test.** This is most important if your sex partner was not treated or if you have a new sex partner.

> ✔ **Quick Tip**
>
> Doctors, local health departments, and STI and family planning clinics have information about STIs. And they can all test you for chlamydia. Don't assume your doctor will test you for chlamydia when you have your Pap test. Take care of yourself by asking for a chlamydia test.

What health problems can result from untreated chlamydia?

Untreated chlamydia can damage a woman's reproductive organs and cause other health problems. Like the disease itself, the damage chlamydia causes is often silent.

For women, untreated chlamydia may lead to these complications:

- **Pelvic Inflammatory Disease (PID):** PID occurs when chlamydia bacteria infect the cells of the cervix, then spread to the uterus, fallopian tubes, and ovaries. PID occurs in up to 40 percent of women with untreated chlamydia. PID can lead to:

    - **Infertility:** You can't get pregnant because the infection scars the fallopian tubes and keeps eggs from being fertilized.

    - **Ectopic Or Tubal Pregnancy:** This happens when a fertilized egg implants outside the uterus. It is a medical emergency.

    - **Chronic Pelvic Pain:** Ongoing pain, most often from scar tissue.

- **Cystitis:** Inflammation of the bladder.

- **HIV/AIDS**: Women who have chlamydia are five times more likely to get HIV, the virus that causes AIDS, from a partner who is infected with it.

For men, untreated chlamydia may lead to: infection and scarring of the urethra, the tube that carries urine from the body; prostatitis, swelling of the prostate gland; infection in the tube that carries sperm from the testes, causing pain and fever; and infertility.

For women and men, untreated chlamydia may lead to: chlamydia bacteria in the throat, if you have oral sex with an infected partner; proctitis, which is an infection of the lining of the rectum, if you have anal sex with an infected partner; and Reiter's syndrome, which causes arthritis, eye redness, and urinary tract problems.

For pregnant women, chlamydia infections may lead to premature delivery. And babies born to infected mothers can get these health problems:

- **Eye Infections (Conjunctivitis, Or Pinkeye):** Symptoms include discharge from the eyes and swollen eyelids. The symptoms most often show up within the first 10 days of life. If left untreated, it can lead to blindness.

- **Pneumonia:** Symptoms include congestion and a cough that keeps getting worse. Both symptoms most often show up within three to six weeks of birth.

How can chlamydia be prevented?

You can take steps to lower your risk of getting chlamydia and other STIs. The following steps work best when used together. No single strategy can protect you from every type of STI.

- **Don't have sex.** The surest way to avoid getting chlamydia or any STI is to practice abstinence. This means not having vaginal, anal, or oral sex.

✤ It's A Fact!!
Eye infections and pneumonia can be treated with antibiotics.

- **Be faithful.** Having sex with only one unaffected partner who only has sex with you will keep you safe from chlamydia and other STIs. Both partners must be faithful all the time to avoid STI exposure. This means you have sex only with each other and no one else. The fewer sex partners you have, the lower your risk of being exposed to chlamydia and other STIs.

- **Use condoms correctly and every time you have sex.** Use condoms for all types of sexual contact, even if penetration does not take place.

- **Know that most methods of birth control—and other methods—will not protect you from chlamydia and other STIs.**

- **Talk with your sex partner(s) about STIs and using condoms before having sex.** Make it clear that you will not have any type of sex at any time without a condom. It's up to you to make sure you are protected. Remember, it's your body!

- **Get tested for STIs.** If either you or your partner has had other sexual partners in the past, get tested for STIs before becoming sexually active.

- **Learn the symptoms of chlamydia.** But remember, chlamydia often has no symptoms. Seek medical help right away if you think you may have chlamydia or another STI.

- **Have regular checkups and pelvic exams—even if you think you're healthy.** During the checkup, your doctor will ask you a lot of questions about your lifestyle, including your sex life. This might seem too personal to share. But answering honestly is the only way your doctor is sure to give you the care you need.

Chapter 56

Gonorrhea

What is gonorrhea?

Gonorrhea is a common sexually transmitted infection (STI). It's caused by a type of bacteria that can grow in warm, moist areas of the reproductive tract, like the cervix, uterus, and fallopian tubes in women. It can grow in the urethra in men and women. It can also grow in the mouth, throat, eyes, and anus.

How do you get gonorrhea?

You can get gonorrhea during vaginal, oral, or anal sex with an infected partner. A man does not need to ejaculate to pass the infection or to become infected. Touching infected sex organs, like the vagina or penis, and then touching your eyes can cause an eye infection. Gonorrhea is not spread by shaking hands or sitting on toilet seats.

Gonorrhea also can be passed from a pregnant woman to her baby during delivery. In babies, gonorrhea infection can cause blindness, joint infection, or a life-threatening blood infection.

About This Chapter: Information in this chapter is from "Gonorrhea: Frequently Asked Questions," a publication of the U.S. Department of Health and Human Services, Office on Women's Health, September 2009.

Who is at risk for gonorrhea?

Any sexually active person can be infected with gonorrhea. In the United States, the highest reported rates of infection are among sexually active teenagers, young adults, and African Americans. In 2007, young women had over two times the gonorrhea rate of young men.

What are the symptoms of gonorrhea?

Many women who have gonorrhea do not have symptoms. When a woman does have symptoms, they often appear within 10 days of getting the STI. But symptoms can be so mild or general that they are overlooked or mistaken for something else.

A woman may have some of these symptoms:

- Pain or burning when passing urine

- Vaginal discharge that is yellow or sometimes bloody

- Bleeding between menstrual periods

- Heavy bleeding with periods

- Pain during sex

✔ **Quick Tip**
If you have any symptoms of gonorrhea, stop having sex and see a doctor right away. Women with gonorrhea are at risk of developing serious health problems, whether or not there are symptoms.

For women and men, symptoms of an anal infection can include discharge, soreness, bleeding, or itching of the anus, and painful bowel movements. Infections in the throat may cause a sore throat but usually cause no symptoms. With an eye infection, symptoms may include redness, itching, or discharge from the eye.

For men, symptoms can include the following:

- Discharge from or pain inside the penis

- Pain or burning while passing urine

- Painful or swollen testicles

> **✔ Quick Tip**
>
> If your partner has any symptoms of gonorrhea, stop having sex and ask your doctor about testing for both of you.

Are there tests for gonorrhea?

Yes. There are three types of tests for gonorrhea:

- **Swab Sample:** A swab sample from the part of the body likely to be infected (cervix, urethra, penis, rectum, or throat) can be sent to a lab for testing.

- **Urine Test:** Gonorrhea in the cervix or urethra can be diagnosed with a urine sample sent to a lab.

- **Gram Stain:** This is done right in a clinic or doctor's office. A sample from the urethra or a cervix is placed on a slide and stained with dye. It allows the doctor to see the bacteria under a microscope. This test works better for men than for women.

How is gonorrhea treated?

Antibiotics are used to cure gonorrhea. But more and more people are becoming infected with types of gonorrhea that do not respond well to drugs. This problem is making it harder to treat gonorrhea. Many people who have gonorrhea also have chlamydia. So, doctors often give medicine to treat both STIs at the same time. For treatment to work, you must finish all the medicine that your doctor gives you, even if the symptoms go away. If symptoms don't go away after treatment, see your doctor. Although treatment can cure the infection, it cannot fix any permanent damage done by the infection. Also, you can get gonorrhea again if you have sex with an infected person.

> **✔ Quick Tip**
>
> Talk to your doctor about getting tested if you have any symptoms of gonorrhea, if you think you or your partner could have it, or if you know your partner has it. If you are tested for gonorrhea, you also should be tested for other STIs, including chlamydia, syphilis, and HIV.

What happens if gonorrhea isn't treated?

Gonorrhea that is not treated can cause these serious problems in women:

- **Pelvic Inflammatory Disease (PID):** PID is an infection of a woman's reproductive organs above the cervix, such as the fallopian tubes and ovaries. Untreated gonorrhea is a common cause of PID. PID can lead to infertility, pregnancy problems, and pelvic pain. Some women have no symptoms of PID, and the damage caused by PID cannot be fixed. This is why finding out about and treating gonorrhea is so important.

- **Widespread Infection:** Infection can spread to other parts of the body, like the blood, joints, or heart.

- **Human Immunodeficiency Virus (HIV):** Increased risk of getting HIV or spreading HIV.

Can gonorrhea cause problems during pregnancy?

Yes. A pregnant woman with untreated gonorrhea has a higher risk of miscarriage, preterm birth, or having her water break too early. Also, her baby could get the infection while passing through the birth canal during delivery. This can cause blindness, joint infection, or a life-threatening blood infection in the baby. Treating the newborn's eyes with medicine right after birth can prevent eye infection. Treatment of gonorrhea as soon as it is found in pregnant women will lower the risk of these problems. All sex partners of pregnant women with gonorrhea must also be treated. If you are pregnant, ask your doctor about testing for STIs, including gonorrhea. Testing is simple, and treatment usually cures the infection and prevents problems for the baby.

How can I keep from getting gonorrhea?

There are steps you can take to lower your risk of getting gonorrhea:

- **Don't have sex.** The surest way to keep from getting gonorrhea is to practice abstinence. This means not having vaginal, oral, or anal sex.

- **Be faithful.** Having a sexual relationship with one partner who has been tested for gonorrhea and is not infected is another way to lower your risk of getting infected. Be faithful to each other. This means you only have sex with each other and no one else.

- **Use condoms.** Use condoms the right way and every time you have vaginal, anal, or oral sex. Because a man does not need to ejaculate to give or get gonorrhea, make sure to put on the condom before the penis touches the vagina, mouth, or anus. Use a new condom if you want to have sex again or in a different way. For vaginal sex, use a latex male condom or a female polyurethane condom. For anal sex, use a latex male condom. For oral sex use a male latex condom. A dental dam might offer some protection during oral sex (mouth to vagina/anus).

- **Know that some methods of birth control, like birth control pills, shots, implants, or diaphragms, will not protect you from STIs, including gonorrhea.** If you use one of these methods, be sure to also use a condom correctly every time you have sex.

- **Talk with your sex partner(s) about STIs and using condoms.** It's up to you to make sure you are protected. Remember, it's your body!

- **Talk frankly with your doctor and your sex partner(s) about any STIs you or your partner has or has had.** Talk about symptoms, such as sores or discharge. Try not to be embarrassed. Being honest could prevent serious health problems.

- **Have a yearly pelvic exam.** Ask your doctor if you should be tested for gonorrhea or other STIs, and how often you should be retested. Testing for many STIs is simple and often can be done during your checkup. The sooner gonorrhea is found the more likely it can be cured before permanent damage is done.

- **If you are pregnant, get tested for gonorrhea.** Get tested as soon as you think you may be pregnant.

I just found out I have gonorrhea. What should I do?

- **Finish all the medicine that your doctor gives you.** Even if the symptoms go away, you still need to finish treatment. If symptoms continue after treatment, see your doctor.

- **Talk with your sex partner(s).** Your sex partner(s) should get tested and treated for gonorrhea, even if they don't have any symptoms.

- **Avoid sexual contact until you and your partner(s) have been treated and cured.** People who have had gonorrhea and were treated can get infected again if they have sexual contact with a person who has gonorrhea.

- **Once you have been treated and cured, take steps to lower your risk from getting gonorrhea again.**

Chapter 57

Syphilis

What is syphilis?

Syphilis is a sexually transmitted infection (STI) caused by bacteria. It progresses in stages. Syphilis is easy to cure in its early stages. But without treatment, it can hurt your body's organs, leading to severe illness and even death.

How is syphilis spread?

Syphilis is spread through direct contact with a syphilis sore or rash during vaginal, anal, or oral sex. The bacteria can enter the body through the penis, anus, vagina, mouth, or through broken skin. An infected pregnant woman can also pass the disease to her unborn child. Syphilis is not spread by contact with toilet seats, doorknobs, swimming pools, hot tubs, bathtubs, shared clothing, or eating utensils.

What are the symptoms of syphilis?

Each stage of syphilis has different symptoms. A person infected with syphilis can pass it to others during the first two stages.

About This Chapter: Information in this chapter is from "Syphilis: Frequently Asked Questions," a publication of the U.S. Department of Health and Human Services, Office on Women's Health, July 2009.

Primary Stage: A single sore called a chancre appears in the first or primary stage. Sometimes, more than one sore appears. The time between infection with syphilis and the start of the chancre can range between 10 to 90 days (21 days average). The chancre is usually firm, round, small, and painless. It appears at the spot where the infection entered the body, such as the vulva, vagina, cervix, tongue, lips, or other parts of the body. In this stage, syphilis can be passed to others through contact with the chancre during vaginal, anal, or oral sex. The chancre lasts three to six weeks and heals with or without treatment. If the infection is not treated, it moves to the secondary stage.

Secondary Stage: The secondary stage can start as the chancre is healing or a few weeks after it has healed. It typically starts with a rash on one or more areas of the body. Some or all of these symptoms can appear:

- Skin rash with rough, red, or reddish-brown spots both on the palms of the hands and bottoms of the feet

- Sores on the throat, mouth, or cervix

- Fever

- Swollen glands

- Sore throat

- Patchy hair loss

- Headaches and muscle aches

- Weight loss

- Tiredness

> ♣ **It's A Fact!!**
> The rash associated with syphilis usually does not itch. Rashes on other parts of the body may not look the same.

In this stage, the infection can be passed to others through contact with open sores or rash during vaginal, anal, or oral sex. Rash and other symptoms will go away with or without treatment. But without treatment, the infection will move to the latent and possibly late stages of disease.

Latent Stage: The latent, or hidden, stage starts when symptoms from the first and second stages go away. The latent stage can last for many, many years. During this stage, the infection lives in the body even though there are no signs or symptoms. The infection cannot be passed to others during the latent stage.

✔ Quick Tip

You will only reach the late stage of syphilis if you do not receive treatment earlier. If you have syphilis, get treated as soon as possible to avoid the problems of late-stage syphilis.

Sometimes, symptoms from the secondary phase come back. If this happens, the infection can be passed to others until the symptoms go away again. Without treatment, the infection will advance to the late stage in some people.

Late Stage: About 15 percent of people with untreated syphilis will advance to the late stage. This can happen within a few years or as many as 20 years or more after first becoming infected. In the late stage, the disease can hurt your organs, including the brain, nerves, eyes, heart, blood vessels, liver, bones, and joints. This damage can lead to nerve problems, paralysis, blindness, dementia, and other health problems. Some people may die from the disease.

How do I find out if I have syphilis?

A doctor can tell if you have syphilis. These are two of the most common ways:

- Taking a sample of your blood and sending it to a lab for testing.

- Looking at the fluid from a syphilis sore under a special type of microscope. This can only be done during primary and secondary stages, when a sore is present.

How is syphilis treated?

Penicillin (an antibiotic) is the preferred drug to treat syphilis at all stages. The dose and length of treatment depends on the stage of syphilis and symptoms of the disease. For people who are allergic to penicillin, other drugs might work during the first and second stages. But they cannot be used by pregnant women. In late syphilis, treatment will prevent further harm, but damage already done to body organs cannot be reversed.

❖ **It's A Fact!!**
Treatment does not protect you from getting syphilis again. You can get syphilis again after being cured if you are exposed to it.

What happens if syphilis isn't treated?

Without treatment, syphilis can lead to severe illness and even death. Having syphilis also increases your risk of getting or giving human immunodeficiency virus (HIV), the disease that causes acquired immune deficiency syndrome (AIDS). The open sores caused by syphilis make it easier for HIV to spread through sexual contact. If you have syphilis, you are thought to be two to five times more likely to get HIV if exposed. Untreated syphilis also can cause problems during pregnancy.

Can syphilis cause problems during pregnancy?

Yes. Pregnant women can pass syphilis to their babies during pregnancy and childbirth. It can cause miscarriage, stillbirth, or death soon after birth. An infected baby may be born without signs of disease. However, if not treated right away, the baby may have serious problems within a few weeks. Babies born with syphilis may develop skin sores, rashes, fever, jaundice, anemia, or a swollen liver and spleen. Untreated babies may become developmentally delayed, have seizures, or die.

All pregnant women should be tested for syphilis. Pregnant women with syphilis are treated right away with penicillin. For women who are allergic to penicillin, no other drugs are available for treatment. So, doctors try to help women with this allergy become less sensitive to the penicillin so it can be used. Penicillin will prevent passing syphilis to the baby. But women who are treated during the second half of pregnancy still are at risk of premature labor and problems with the unborn baby.

How can I keep from getting syphilis?

There are steps you can take to lower your risk of getting syphilis:

- **Don't have sex.** The surest way to keep from getting syphilis is to practice abstinence. This means not having vaginal, oral, or anal sex.

- **Be faithful.** Having a sexual relationship with one partner who has been tested for syphilis and is not infected is another way to lower your risk of getting infected. Be faithful to each other. This means you only have sex with each other and no one else.

- **Use condoms.** Syphilis sores can occur in places that are covered by a condom, as well as areas that are not covered. So, using a condom the right way and every time you have vaginal, anal, or oral sex might lower your risk. For vaginal sex, use a latex male condom or a female polyurethane condom. For anal sex, use a latex male condom. For oral sex use a male latex condom. A dental dam might offer some protection during oral sex (mouth to vagina/anus).

- **Know that some methods of birth control, like birth control pills, shots, implants, or diaphragms, will not protect you from STIs, including syphilis.** If you use one of these methods, be sure to also use a latex condom every time you have sex.

- **Talk with your sex partner(s) about STIs and using condoms.** It's up to you to make sure you are protected. Remember, it's your body!

- **Talk frankly with your doctor and your sex partner(s) about any STIs you or your partner has or has had.** Talk about symptoms, such as sores or discharge. Try not to be embarrassed. Your doctor is there to help you with any and all health problems. Also, being open with your partners can help you protect your health and the health of others.

- **Have a yearly pelvic exam.** Ask your doctor if you should be tested for syphilis or other STIs, and how often you should be retested. Testing for many STIs is simple and often can be done during your checkup. The sooner syphilis is found, the more likely it can be cured quickly and easily.

- **Avoid using drugs or drinking too much alcohol.** These activities may lead to risky sexual behavior such as not wearing a condom.

Who should get tested for syphilis?

Ask your doctor about getting tested for syphilis if these characteristics apply to you:

- You have symptoms and signs of syphilis.

- You think you might have been exposed to someone with syphilis.

- You are pregnant. All pregnant women should be tested for syphilis at their first prenatal checkup. Some pregnant women should be tested again, later in the pregnancy. Ask your doctor about retesting.

- Your or your partner's sexual behavior puts you at risk for STIs (such as having sex with multiple partners, having unprotected sex, or having sex with men who have sex with men). Ask your doctor how often you should be retested.

- You have another STI.

I just found out I have syphilis. What should I do?

- **Follow all your doctor's treatment orders.** Even if the symptoms go away, you still need to finish treatment. If symptoms continue after treatment, see your doctor.

- **Avoid any sexual activity while you are being treated for syphilis.** Don't have sexual contact until the syphilis sores are completely healed.

- **Tell your sex partner(s).** Your sex partner(s) should get tested for syphilis and treated if needed.

- **After you have completed treatment for syphilis, get retested after six months and twelve months.** Some doctors recommend more frequent follow-up tests.

- **Get tested for HIV.** If your test result is negative, ask your doctor if you need to be retested and when.

- **Once you have been treated and cured, take steps to lower your risk from getting syphilis again.**

Chapter 58

Chancroid

Chancroid is a bacterial disease that is spread only through sexual contact.

Causes

Chancroid is caused by a type of bacteria called *Haemophilus ducreyi*.

The disease is found mainly in developing and third world countries. Only a small number of cases are diagnosed in the United States each year. Most people in the U.S. diagnosed with chancroid have traveled outside the country to areas where the disease is known to occur frequently.

Symptoms

Within one day–two weeks after getting chancroid, a person will get a small bump in the genitals. The bump becomes an ulcer within a day of its appearance. The ulcer:

- ranges in size from 1/8 inch to 2 inches across
- is painful
- is soft
- has sharply defined borders

About This Chapter: Information in this chapter is from "Chancroid," © 2010 A.D.A.M., Inc. Reprinted with permission.

- has irregular or ragged borders

- has a base that is covered with a grey or yellowish-grey material

- has a base that bleeds easily if banged or scraped

Common locations in men are:

- foreskin (prepuce)

- groove behind the head of the penis (coronal sulcus)

- shaft of the penis

- head of the penis (glans)

- opening of the penis (urethral meatus)

- scrotum

❖ **It's A Fact!!**
Uncircumcised men are at much higher risk than circumcised men for getting chancroid from an infected partner. Chancroid is a risk factor for the human immunodeficiency virus (HIV) virus.

In women the most common location for ulcers is the outer lips of the vagina (labia majora). "Kissing ulcers" may develop. These are ulcers that occur on opposite surfaces of the labia. Other areas such as the inner vagina lips (labia minora), the area between the genitals and the anus (perineal area), and inner thighs may also be involved. The most common symptoms in women are pain with urination and intercourse.

Approximately half of the people infected with a chancroid will develop enlarged inguinal lymph nodes, the nodes located in the fold between the leg and the lower abdomen.

Half of those who have swelling of the inguinal lymph nodes will progress to a point where the nodes break through the skin, producing draining abscesses. The swollen lymph nodes and abscesses are often referred to as buboes.

❖ **It's A Fact!!**
About half of infected men have only a single ulcer. Women often have four or more ulcers. The ulcers appear in specific locations.

❖ It's A Fact!!
The chancroid ulcer may look like a chancre, the typical sore of primary syphilis.

Exams And Tests

Chancroid is diagnosed by looking at the ulcer(s) and checking for swollen lymph nodes. There are no blood tests for chancroid.

Treatment

The infection is treated with antibiotics, including azithromycin, ceftriaxone, ciprofloxacin, and erythromycin. Large lymph node swellings need to be drained, either with a needle or local surgery.

Outlook (Prognosis)

Chancroid can get better on its own. However, some people may have months of painful ulcers and draining. Antibiotic treatment usually clears up the lesions quickly with very little scarring.

Possible Complications

Complications include urethral fistulas and scars on the foreskin of the penis in uncircumcised males. Patients with chancroid should also be checked for syphilis, HIV, and genital herpes.

When To Contact A Medical Professional

Call for an appointment with your health care provider if you have symptoms of chancroid. Also call if you have had sexual contact with a person known to have any STD, or if you have engaged in high-risk sexual practices.

❖ It's A Fact!!
Chancroids in persons with HIV may take much longer to heal.

Prevention

Chancroid is a bacterial infection that is spread by sexual contact with an infected person. Avoiding all forms of sexual activity is the only absolute way to prevent a sexually transmitted disease.

However, safe sex behaviors may reduce your risk. The proper use of condoms, either the male or female type, greatly decreases the risk of catching a sexually transmitted disease. You need to wear the condom from the beginning to the end of each sexual activity.

Chapter 59

Lymphogranuloma Venereum (LGV)

What is LGV?

LGV (Lymphogranuloma venereum) is a sexually transmitted disease (STD) caused by three strains of the bacterium *Chlamydia trachomatis*. The visual signs include genital papule(s) (e.g., raised surfaces or bumps) and/or ulcers, and swelling of the lymph glands in the genital area. LGV may also produce rectal ulcers, bleeding, pain, and discharge, especially among those who practice receptive anal intercourse. Genital lesions caused by LGV can be mistaken for other ulcerative STDs such as syphilis, genital herpes, and chancroid. Complications of untreated LGV may include enlargement and ulcerations of the external genitalia and lymphatic obstruction, which may lead to elephantiasis of the genitalia.

How common is LGV?

Signs and symptoms associated with rectal infection can be mistakenly thought to be caused by ulcerative colitis. While the frequency of LGV infection is thought to be rare in industrialized countries, its identification is not always obvious, so the number of cases of LGV in the United States is unknown. However, outbreaks in the Netherlands and other European countries among men who have sex with men (MSM) have raised concerns about cases of LGV in the U.S.

About This Chapter: Information in this chapter is from "LGV," a fact sheet from the Centers for Disease Control and Prevention, December 2007.

How do people get LGV?

LGV is passed from person to person through direct contact with lesions, ulcers, or other areas where the bacteria is located. Transmission of the organism occurs during sexual penetration (vaginal, oral, or anal) and may also occur via skin-to-skin contact. The likelihood of LGV infection following an exposure is unknown, but it is considered less infectious than some other STDs. A person who has had sexual contact with a LGV-infected partner within 60 days of symptom onset should be examined, tested for urethral or cervical chlamydial infection, and treated with doxycycline twice daily for seven days.

What are the signs and symptoms?

LGV can be difficult to diagnose. Typically, the primary lesion produced by LGV is a small genital or rectal lesion, which can ulcerate at the site of transmission after an incubation period of 3–30 days. These ulcers may remain undetected within the urethra, vagina, or rectum.

How is LGV diagnosed?

Because of limitations in a commercially available test, diagnosis is primarily based on clinical findings. Direct identification of the bacteria from a lesion or site of the infection may be possible through testing for chlamydia but this would not indicate if the chlamydia infection is LGV. However, the usual chlamydia tests that are available have not been approved by the U.S. Food and Drug Administration (FDA) for testing rectal specimens. In a patient with rectal signs or symptoms suspicious for LGV, a health care provider can collect a specimen and send the sample to his/her state health department for referral to Centers for Disease Control and Prevention (CDC), which is working with state and local health departments to test specimens and validate diagnostic methods for LGV.

❖ It's A Fact!!
As with other STDs that cause ulcers, LGV may facilitate transmission and acquisition of human immunodeficiency virus (HIV).

What is the treatment for LGV?

There is no vaccine against the bacteria. LGV can be treated with three weeks of antibiotics.

CDC STD Treatment Guidelines recommend the use of doxycyline twice a day for 21 days. An alternative treatment is erythromycin base or azithromycin. The health care provider will determine which is best.

✤ **It's A Fact!!**

Doxycycline is not recommended for use in pregnant women. Pregnant and lactating women should be treated with erythromycin. Azythromycin may prove useful for treatment of LGV in pregnancy, but no published data are available regarding its safety and efficacy. A health care provider (like a doctor or nurse) can discuss treatment options with patients.

If you have been treated for LGV, you should notify any sex partners you had sex with within 60 days of the symptom onset so they can be evaluated and treated. This will reduce the risk that your partners will develop symptoms and/or serious complications of LGV. It will reduce your risk of becoming reinfected as well as reduce the risk of ongoing transmission in the community. You and all of your sex partners should avoid sex until you have completed treatment for the infection and your symptoms and your partners' symptoms have disappeared.

Persons with both LGV and HIV infection should receive the same LGV treatment as those who are HIV negative. Prolonged therapy may be required, and delay in resolution of symptoms may occur among persons with HIV.

How can LGV be prevented?

The surest way to avoid transmission of sexually transmitted diseases is to abstain from sexual contact, or to be in a long-term mutually monogamous relationship with a partner who has been tested and is asymptomatic and uninfected.

✤ **It's A Fact!!**

Having had LGV and completing treatment does not prevent reinfection. Effective treatment is available and it is important that persons suspected of having LGV be treated as if they have it. Persons who are treated for LGV treatment should abstain from sexual contact until the infection is cleared.

Male latex condoms, when used consistently and correctly, may reduce the risk of LGV transmission. Genital ulcer diseases can occur in male or female genital areas that may or may not be covered (protected by the condom).

Chapter 60

Genital Herpes

What is genital herpes?

Genital herpes is a sexually transmitted infection (STI) caused by the herpes simplex viruses type 1 (HSV-1) or type 2 (HSV-2). Most genital herpes is caused by HSV-2. HSV-1 can cause genital herpes. But it more commonly causes infections of the mouth and lips, called fever blisters.

Most people have no or few symptoms from herpes infection. When symptoms do occur, they usually appear as one or more blisters on or around the genitals or rectum. The blisters break, leaving tender sores that may take up to four weeks to heal. Another outbreak can appear weeks or months later. But it almost always is less severe and shorter than the first outbreak.

Although the infection can stay in the body forever, the outbreaks tend to become less severe and occur less often over time. You can pass genital herpes to someone else even when you have no symptoms.

How common is genital herpes?

Genital herpes is common. At least 45 million Americans age 12 and older have genital herpes. Genital HSV-2 infection is more common in women than

About This Chapter: Information in this chapter is from "Genital Herpes: Frequently Asked Questions," a publication of the U.S. Department of Health and Human Services, Office on Women's Health, August 2009.

men. About one in four women have HSV-2 infection compared to almost one in eight men. This is because women can get genital herpes and some other STIs more easily than men.

How is genital herpes spread?

You can get genital herpes through genital-genital contact or genital-oral contact with someone who has herpes infection. The virus is most easily spread through contact with open sores. But you also can get the virus from skin that does not appear to have a sore. You can become infected with the herpes virus without having intercourse.

What are the symptoms of genital herpes?

The symptoms of genital herpes vary from person to person. Most people with genital herpes are not aware they are infected. But, if symptoms do occur with the first outbreak, they can be severe. Genital herpes infection also can be severe and long lasting in people whose immune systems don't work properly, such as people with human immunodeficiency virus (HIV).

The first outbreak usually happens within two weeks of having sexual contact with an infected person, and symptoms can last from two to three weeks. Early symptoms of the first outbreak can include: itching or burning feeling in the genital or anal area; flu-like symptoms, including fever; swollen glands; pain in the legs, buttocks, or genital area; vaginal discharge; and a feeling of pressure in the area below the stomach.

Within a few days, sores show up where the virus has entered the body, such as on the mouth, penis, or vagina. Sores can also show up on a woman's cervix or in the urinary passage in men. The sores are small red bumps that may turn into blisters or painful open sores. Over a period of days, the sores become crusted and then heal without scarring. Sometimes with the first outbreak, a second crop of sores appear and flu-like symptoms occur again.

Some people have no symptoms. Or they might mistake mild sores for insect bites or something else. Yet even without symptoms, a person can still pass the herpes virus to others. So, if you have signs of herpes, see your doctor to find out if you are infected.

Can genital herpes come back?

Yes. Herpes symptoms can come and go, but the virus stays inside your body even after all signs of the infection have gone away. In most people, the virus becomes active from time to time, creating an outbreak. Some people have herpes virus outbreaks only once or twice. People who have a first outbreak can expect to have four or five outbreaks within a year. Over time, the outbreaks tend to occur less often and be less severe. Experts don't know what causes the virus to become active. Some women say the virus comes back when they are sick, under stress, out in the sun, or having their period.

> ✔ **Quick Tip**
>
> If you have herpes, do not have any sexual activity with an uninfected partner when you have sores or other symptoms of herpes. Even if you don't have symptoms, you can still pass the virus to others.

How do I know for sure if I have genital herpes?

Doctors can diagnose genital herpes by looking at visible sores if the outbreak is typical and by taking a sample from the sore for testing in a lab. Some cases of herpes are harder to diagnose, especially between outbreaks. Blood tests that look for antibodies to HSV-1 or HSV-2 can help to detect herpes infection in people without symptoms or between outbreaks.

What is the treatment for genital herpes?

Genital herpes cannot be cured; the virus will always be in your body. But the antiviral drugs acyclovir, valacyclovir, and famciclovir can shorten outbreaks and make them less severe, or stop them from happening. Valacyclovir (brand name Valtrex) also can lower your risk of passing the infection to someone else.

> ✔ **Quick Tip**
>
> Depending on your needs, your doctor can give you drugs to take right after getting outbreak symptoms or drugs to take on a regular basis to try to stop outbreaks from happening. Talk to your doctor about treatment options.

During outbreaks, these steps can speed healing and help keep the infection from spreading to other sites of the body or to other people:

- Keep the infected area clean and dry.

- Try not to touch the sores.

- Wash hands after contact.

- Avoid sexual contact from the time you first notice symptoms until the sores have healed.

> **❖ It's A Fact!!**
>
> There is no cure for genital herpes. Once you have the virus, it stays in your body and there is a chance that you will have outbreaks. Medicine can shorten outbreaks and stop them from happening.

Can genital herpes cause other problems?

Genital herpes infection usually does not cause serious health problems in healthy adults. People whose immune systems don't work properly, such as people with HIV, can have severe outbreaks that are long lasting. Sometimes, people with normal immune systems can get herpes infection in the eye. But this is less common with HSV-2 infection.

What can I do to keep from getting genital herpes?

There are things you can do to lower your risk of getting genital herpes:

- **Don't have sex.** The surest way to prevent any STI, including genital herpes, is to practice abstinence, or not having vaginal, oral, or anal sex. Keep in mind, you can get genital herpes from close contact other than sexual intercourse.

- **Be faithful.** Having a sexual relationship with one partner who has been tested for herpes and is not infected is another way to lower your risk of getting infected. Be faithful to each other, meaning that you only have sex with each other and no one else.

- **Use condoms.** Use condoms correctly and every time you have any type of sex. For vaginal sex, use a latex male condom or a female polyurethane condom. For anal sex, use a latex male condom. For oral sex, use a dental dam. Keep in mind that condoms may not cover all infected areas, so you can still get herpes even if you use a condom.

- **Know that some methods of birth control, like birth control pills, shots, implants, or diaphragms, will not protect you from STIs.** If you use one of these methods, be sure to also use a latex condom or dental dam correctly and every time you have sex.

- **Talk with your sex partner(s) about STIs and using condoms.** It's up to you to make sure you are protected. Remember, it's your body!

- **Talk frankly with your doctor and your sex partner(s) about any STIs you or your partner has or has had.** If you feel embarrassed, try to put this aside. Your doctor is there to help you with any and all health problems. Also, being open with your partners can help you protect your health and the health of others.

- **Know the symptoms.** Learn the common symptoms of genital herpes and other STIs. Do not have oral-genital contact if you or your partner has any signs of oral herpes, such as a fever blister. Seek medical help right away if you think you may have genital herpes or another STI. Don't have sexual contact until you have seen your doctor.

What should I do if I have genital herpes?

- See your doctor for testing and treatment right away.

- Follow your doctor's orders and finish all the medicine that you are given. Even if the symptoms go away, you still need to finish all of the medicine.

- Avoid having any sexual activity while you are being treated for genital herpes and while you have any symptoms of an outbreak.

- Be sure to tell your sexual partners, so they can be tested.

- Remember that genital herpes is a lifelong disease. Even though you may have long periods with no symptoms, you can still pass the virus to another person. Talk with your doctor about what you can do to have fewer future outbreaks, and how to prevent passing the virus to another person.

What should I do if my partner has genital herpes?

- Get tested to find out if you also are infected with the herpes virus.

- Avoid having any sexual activity while your partner is being treated for a genital herpes outbreak or if your partner has symptoms of an outbreak, such as open sores.

- Use condoms correctly and every time you have sex to lower your risk of becoming infected.

- Talk to your partner about using daily suppressive therapy to reduce the number of outbreaks and lower the risk of infecting you with the virus.

Chapter 61

Human Papillomavirus (HPV)

What is genital HPV infection?

Genital human papillomavirus (also called HPV) is the most common sexually transmitted infection (STI). There are more than 40 HPV types that can infect the genital areas of males and females. These HPV types can also infect the mouth and throat. Most people who become infected with HPV do not even know they have it.

What are the signs, symptoms, and potential health problems of HPV?

Most people with HPV do not develop symptoms or health problems from it. In 90% of cases, the body's immune system clears HPV naturally within two years. But sometimes, certain types of HPV can cause genital warts in males and females. Rarely, these types can also cause warts in the throat—a condition called recurrent respiratory papillomatosis or RRP.

Other HPV types can cause cervical cancer. These types can also cause other, less common but serious cancers, including cancers of the vulva, vagina, penis, anus, and head and neck (tongue, tonsils, and throat).

About This Chapter: Information in this chapter is from "Genital HPV Infection," a fact sheet from the Centers for Disease Control and Prevention, November 2009.

These are common signs and symptoms of HPV-related problems:

- **Genital warts usually appear as a small bump or groups of bumps in the genital area.** They can be small or large, raised or flat, or shaped like a cauliflower. Health care providers can diagnose warts by looking at the genital area during an office visit. Warts can appear within weeks or months after sexual contact with an infected partner—even if the infected partner has no signs of genital warts. If left untreated, genital warts might go away, remain unchanged, or increase in size or number. They will not turn into cancer.

> ❖ **It's A Fact!!**
> The types of HPV that can cause genital warts are not the same as the types that can cause cancer. There is no way to know which people who get HPV will go on to develop cancer or other health problems.

- **Cervical cancer usually does not have symptoms until it is quite advanced.** For this reason, it is important for women to get regular screening for cervical cancer. Screening tests can find early signs of disease so that problems can be treated early, before they ever turn into cancer.

- **Other HPV-related cancers might not have signs or symptoms until they are advanced and hard to treat.** These include cancers of the vulva, vagina, penis, anus, and head and neck.

- **RRP causes warts to grow in the throat.** It can sometimes block the airway, causing a hoarse voice or troubled breathing.

How do people get HPV?

HPV is passed on through genital contact, most often during vaginal and anal sex. HPV may also be passed on during oral sex and genital-to-genital contact. HPV can be passed on between straight and same-sex partners—even when the infected partner has no signs or symptoms.

A person can have HPV even if years have passed since he or she had sexual contact with an infected person. Most infected persons do not realize they are infected or that they are passing the virus on to a sex partner. It is also possible to get more than one type of HPV.

Very rarely, a pregnant woman with genital HPV can pass HPV to her baby during delivery. In these cases, the child can develop RRP.

How does HPV cause genital warts and cancer?

HPV can cause normal cells on infected skin to turn abnormal. Most of the time, you cannot see or feel these cell changes. In most cases, the body fights off HPV naturally and the infected cells then go back to normal. But in cases when the body does not fight off HPV, HPV can cause visible changes in the form of genital warts or cancer. Warts can appear within weeks or months after getting HPV. Cancer often takes years to develop after getting HPV.

How can people prevent HPV?

There are several ways that people can lower their chances of getting HPV:

- **Vaccines can protect males and females against some of the most common types of HPV.** These vaccines are given in three shots. It is important to get all three doses to get the best protection. The vaccines are most effective when given before a person's first sexual contact, when he or she could be exposed to HPV.

- **Girls And Women:** Two vaccines (Cervarix and Gardasil) are available to protect females against the types of HPV that cause most cervical cancers. One of these vaccines (Gardasil) also protects against most genital warts. Both vaccines are recommended for 11- and 12-year-old girls and for females 13 through 26 years of age who did not get any or all of the shots when they were younger. These vaccines can also be given to girls as young as nine years of age. It is recommended that females get the same vaccine brand for all three doses, whenever possible.

> **❖ It's A Fact!!**
>
> Certain populations are at higher risk for some HPV-related health problems. This includes gay and bisexual men and people with weak immune systems, including those who have human immunodeficiency virus /acquired immune deficiency syndrome (HIV/AIDS).

- **Boys And Men:** One available vaccine (Gardasil) protects males against most genital warts. This vaccine is available for boys and men, nine through 26 years of age.

- **For those who choose to be sexually active, condoms may lower the risk of HPV.** To be most effective, they should be used with every sex act, from start to finish. Condoms may also lower the risk of developing HPV-related diseases, such as genital warts and cervical cancer. But HPV can infect areas that are not covered by a condom—so condoms may not fully protect against HPV.

- **People can also lower their chances of getting HPV by being in a faithful relationship with one partner, limiting their number of sex partners, and choosing a partner who has had no or few prior sex partners.**

How can people prevent HPV-related diseases?

There are ways to prevent the possible health effects of HPV, including the two most common problems, genital warts and cervical cancer.

- **Preventing Genital Warts:** A vaccine (Gardasil) is available to protect against most genital warts in males and females.

- **Preventing Cervical Cancer:** There are two vaccines (Cervarix and Gardasil) that can protect women against most cervical cancers. Cervical cancer can also be prevented with routine cervical cancer screening and follow-up of abnormal results. The Pap test can find abnormal cells on the cervix so that they can be removed before cancer develops. An HPV deoxyribonucleic acid (DNA) test, which can find HPV on a woman's cervix, may also be used with a Pap test in certain cases. Even women who got the vaccine when they were younger need regular cervical cancer screening because the vaccine does not protect against all cervical cancers.

- **Preventing Anal And Penile Cancers:** There is no approved screening test to find early signs of penile or anal cancer.

- **Preventing Head And Neck Cancers:** There is no approved test to find early signs of head and neck cancer, but tests are available by specialized doctors for persons with possible symptoms of these cancers.

Is there a test for HPV?

The HPV tests on the market are only used to help screen for cervical cancer. There is no general test for men or women to check one's overall HPV status, nor is there an HPV test to find HPV on the genitals or in the mouth or throat. But HPV usually goes away on its own, without causing health problems. So an HPV infection that is found today will most likely not be there a year or two from now.

Is there a treatment for HPV or related diseases?

There is no treatment for the virus itself, but there are treatments for the diseases that HPV can cause:

- **Visible genital warts can be removed by the patient him- or herself with medications.** They can also be treated by a health care provider. Some people choose not to treat warts, but to see if they disappear on their own. No one treatment is better than another.

- **Cervical cancer is most treatable when it is diagnosed and treated early.** But women who get routine Pap tests and follow up as needed can identify problems before cancer develops. Prevention is always better than treatment.

- **Other HPV-related cancers are also more treatable when diagnosed and treated early.**

- **RRP can be treated with surgery or medicines.** It can sometimes take many treatments or surgeries over a period of years.

Chapter 62

Hepatitis

What is hepatitis?

Hepatitis means inflammation of the liver. Hepatitis is most often caused by one of several viruses, such as hepatitis A virus, hepatitis B virus, or hepatitis C virus. Toxins, bacterial infections, certain drugs, other diseases, and heavy alcohol use can also cause hepatitis.

What is hepatitis B?

Hepatitis B is a contagious liver disease that results from infection with the hepatitis B virus. It can range in severity from a mild illness lasting a few weeks to a serious, lifelong illness. Hepatitis B can be either acute or chronic. Acute hepatitis B virus infection is a short-term illness that occurs within the first six months after someone is exposed to the hepatitis B virus. Acute infection can—but does not always—lead to chronic infection. Chronic hepatitis B virus infection is a long-term illness that occurs when the hepatitis B virus remains in a person's body.

About This Chapter: Information in this chapter is from "Hepatitis B: General Information," a publication of the Centers for Disease Control and Prevention, Publication No. 21-1073, June 2010. The chapter also includes information from "Hepatitis C: General Information," a publication of the Centers for Disease Control and Prevention, Publication No. 21-1075, June 2010.

How common is hepatitis B in the United States?

The number of acute hepatitis B virus infections has been declining each year, with an estimated 46,000 new infections in 2006. Many experts believe this decline is a result of widespread vaccination of children. However, up to 1.4 million people may have chronic hepatitis B, many of whom are unaware of their infection.

❖ It's A Fact!!
The best way to prevent hepatitis B is by getting vaccinated.

Source: Centers for Disease Control and Prevention, Publication No. 21-1073, June 2010.

How is hepatitis B spread?

Hepatitis B is usually spread when blood, semen, or another body fluid from a person infected with the hepatitis B virus enters the body of someone who is not infected. This can happen through sexual contact with an infected person or sharing needles, syringes, or other drug-injection equipment. Hepatitis B can also be passed from an infected mother to her baby at birth.

Can hepatitis B be spread through sex?

Yes. In the United States, hepatitis B is most commonly spread through sexual contact. The hepatitis B virus is 50–100 times more infectious than human immunodeficiency virus (HIV) and can be passed through the exchange of body fluids, such as semen, vaginal fluids, and blood.

Who is at risk?

Although anyone can get hepatitis B, some people are at greater risk, such as those to whom these characteristics apply:

❖ It's A Fact!!
Hepatitis B is not spread through breastfeeding, sharing eating utensils, hugging, kissing, holding hands, coughing, or sneezing. Unlike some forms of hepatitis, hepatitis B is not spread by contaminated food or water.

Source: Centers for Disease Control and Prevention, Publication No. 21-1073, June 2010.

✔ Quick Tip
Who should get vaccinated against hepatitis B?

Vaccination is recommended for certain groups, including the following:

- Anyone having sex with an infected partner

- People with multiple sex partners

- Anyone with a sexually transmitted disease

- Men who have sexual contact with other men

- Users of injection drugs

- People who live with someone who is infected

- People with chronic liver disease, end stage renal disease, or HIV infection

- Healthcare and public safety workers exposed to blood

- Residents or staff of facilities for developmentally disabled persons

- Travelers to certain countries

- Infants or children younger than 19 who have not been vaccinated

- Anyone who wants to be protected from hepatitis B

Source: Centers for Disease Control and Prevention, Publication No. 21-1073, June 2010.

- Have sexual contact with an infected person

- Have multiple sex partners

- Have a sexually transmitted disease

- Are men who have sexual encounters with other men

- Inject drugs or share needles, syringes, or other injection equipment

- Live with a person who has hepatitis B

- Are on hemodialysis

- Are exposed to blood on the job

- Are infants born to infected mothers

What are the symptoms of acute hepatitis B?

Not everyone has symptoms with acute hepatitis B, especially young children. Most adults have symptoms that appear within three months of exposure. Symptoms can last from a few weeks to several months and include the following:

- Fever

- Fatigue

- Loss of appetite

- Nausea
- Vomiting
- Abdominal pain
- Dark urine
- Clay-colored bowel movements
- Joint pain
- Jaundice

What are the symptoms of chronic hepatitis B?

Many people with chronic hepatitis B remain symptom free for up to 30 years, but others experience ongoing symptoms similar to those of acute hepatitis B. Chronic hepatitis B is a serious disease that can result in long-term health problems.

How is hepatitis B diagnosed and treated?

Doctors diagnose the infection using one or more blood tests. There is no medication available to treat acute hepatitis B, so doctors usually recommend rest, adequate nutrition, and fluids. People with chronic hepatitis B virus infection should be monitored regularly for signs of liver disease, and some people benefit from treatment with specific medications.

How serious is chronic hepatitis B?

Over time, approximately 15–25 percent of people with chronic hepatitis B develop serious liver problems, including liver damage, cirrhosis, liver failure, and liver cancer. Every year, up to 4,000 people in the United States and more than 600,000 people worldwide die from hepatitis B-related liver disease.

Can hepatitis B be prevented?

Yes. The best way to prevent hepatitis B is by getting vaccinated. For adults, the hepatitis B vaccine series is usually given as three shots during a six-month period. The entire series is needed for long-term protection. However, once a person has been infected with the hepatitis B virus, the vaccine does not provide protection against the disease.

What is hepatitis C?

Hepatitis C is a contagious liver disease that results from infection with the hepatitis C virus. When first infected, a person can develop an acute infection, which can range in severity from a very mild illness with few or no symptoms to a serious condition requiring hospitalization.

Acute hepatitis C is a short-term illness that occurs within the first six months after someone is exposed to the hepatitis C virus. For reasons that are not known, 15–25 percent of people clear the virus without treatment. Approximately 75–85 percent of people who become infected with the hepatitis C virus develop chronic, or lifelong, infection.

Chronic hepatitis C is a long-term illness that occurs when the hepatitis C virus remains in a person's body. Over time, it can lead to serious liver problems, including liver damage, cirrhosis, liver failure, or liver cancer.

How is hepatitis C spread?

Hepatitis C is usually spread when blood from a person infected with the hepatitis C virus enters the body of someone who is not infected. Today, most people become infected with the hepatitis C virus by sharing needles or other equipment to inject drugs. Before widespread screening of the blood supply began in 1992, hepatitis was also commonly spread through blood transfusions and organ transplants. Although rare, outbreaks of hepatitis C have occurred from blood contamination in medical settings.

❖ It's A Fact!!
Can hepatitis C be spread through sex?

Yes, although scientists do not know how frequently this occurs. Rough sex, sex with multiple partners, or having a sexually transmitted disease or HIV appears to increase a person's risk of hepatitis C. There also appears to be an increased risk for sexual transmission of hepatitis C among gay men who are HIV positive.

Source: Centers for Disease Control and Prevention, Publication No. 21-1075, June 2010.

Chapter 63

Molluscum Contagiosum

What is molluscum contagiosum?

Molluscum contagiosum is caused by a virus and usually causes a mild skin disease. The virus affects only the outer (epithelial) layer of skin and does not circulate throughout the body in healthy people.

The virus causes small white, pink, or flesh-colored raised bumps or growths with a dimple or pit in the center. The bumps are usually smooth and firm. In most people, the growths range from about the size of a pinhead to as large as a pencil eraser (2 to 5 millimeters in diameter).

The bumps may appear anywhere on the body, alone or in groups. They are usually painless, although they may be itchy, red, swollen and/or sore.

Who gets molluscum contagiosum?

Molluscum infections occur worldwide but are more common in warm, humid climates and where living conditions are crowded. There is evidence that molluscum infections have been on the rise in the United States since 1966, but these infections are not routinely monitored because they are seldom serious and routinely disappear without treatment.

About This Chapter: Information in this chapter is from "Molluscum (Molluscum Contagiosum): Frequently Asked Questions for Everyone," a publication of the Centers for Disease Control and Prevention, June 2010.

Molluscum is common enough that you should not be surprised if you see someone with it or if someone in your family becomes infected. Although not limited to children, it is most common in children one to 10 years of age. People with weakened immune systems (i.e., human immunodeficiency virus (HIV)-infected persons or persons being treated for cancer) are at higher risk for getting molluscum, and their growths may look different, be larger, and be more difficult to treat.

> ❖ **It's A Fact!!**
> Molluscum usually disappears within six to 12 months without treatment and without leaving scars. Some growths may remain for up to four years.

How do people become infected with the molluscum virus?

The virus that causes molluscum is spread from person to person by touching the affected skin. The virus may also be spread by touching a surface with the virus on it, such as a towel, clothing, or toys. Once someone has the virus, the bumps can spread to other parts of their body by touching or scratching a bump and then touching another part of the body.

Although the virus might be spread by sharing swimming pools, baths, saunas, or other wet and warm environments, this has not been proven. Researchers who have investigated this idea think it is more likely the virus is spread by sharing towels and other items around a pool or sauna than through water.

How would I know if I had molluscum contagiosum?

Only a health care provider can diagnose molluscum infection. If you have any unusual skin irritation, rash, bump(s), or blister(s) that do not disappear in a few days, you should see a health care provider.

> ❖ **It's A Fact!!**
> Molluscum can be spread from one person to another by sexual contact.

If you have molluscum, you will see small white, pink, or flesh-colored raised bumps or growths with a pit or dimple in the center. The bumps are usually smooth and firm.

They can be as small as the head of a pin and as large as a pencil eraser (2 to 5 millimeters in diameter). The growths are usually painless but may become itchy, sore, and red and/or swollen. They may occur anywhere on the body including the face, neck, arms, legs, abdomen, and genital area, alone or in groups. The bumps are rarely found on the palms of the hands or the soles of the feet.

What should I do if I think I have molluscum contagiosum?

If you have any unusual skin irritation, rash, bumps, or blisters that do not disappear in a few days, contact a health care provider. Only a health care professional can diagnose molluscum. He or she will discuss treatment options and how to care for the affected skin.

How can I avoid becoming infected with molluscum?

The best way to avoid getting molluscum is by following good hygiene habits.

- Do not touch, pick, or scratch any skin with bumps or blisters (yours or someone else's).

- Good hand hygiene is the best way to avoid getting many infections including molluscum. By washing your hands frequently you wash away germs picked up from other people or from contaminated surfaces.

✔ Quick Tip

Here's how to wash hands correctly:

1. First wet your hands and apply soap.

2. Next rub your hands vigorously together and scrub all surfaces.

3. Continue for 10–15 seconds. Soap combined with scrubbing action helps dislodge and remove germs.

4. Rinse well and dry your hands.

If I have molluscum, how can I avoid spreading it to others?

- It is important to keep the area with growths clean and covered with clothing or a bandage so that others do not touch the bumps and become infected with molluscum. However, when there is no risk of others coming into contact with your skin, such as at night when you sleep, uncover the bumps to help keep your skin healthy.

- Before participating in sports in which your body will come into contact with another person's body (i.e., wrestling) or shared equipment (swimming pools) cover all growths with clothing or a watertight bandage.

- Do not share towels, clothing, or other personal items.

- Do not shave or have electrolysis on areas with bumps.

- If you have bumps in the genital area, avoid sexual activities until you see a health care provider.

♣ **It's A Fact!!**

Many, but not all, cases of molluscum in adults are caused by sexual contact. Treatment for molluscum is usually recommended if the growths are in the genital area (on or near the penis, vulva, vagina, or anus). If bumps are found in the genital area, it is a good idea to discuss with a health care provider the possibility that you might have another disease that is spread by sexual contact.

♣ **It's A Fact!!**

Molluscum contagiosum is not like herpes viruses, which can remain dormant in your body for long periods and then reappear. So, assuming you do not come in contact with another infected person, once all the molluscum contagiosum bumps go away, you will not develop any new bumps.

How long does the molluscum contagiosum virus stay in my body?

The virus lives only in the skin and once the growths are gone, the virus is gone and you cannot spread the virus to others.

How is molluscum treated?

You should discuss all treatment options with a health care provider. Usually no treatment is needed because the bumps disappear by themselves within six to 12 months, although this may take up to four years.

Cryotherapy (freezing the molluscum growth) is one treatment option. This is the same way that warts are removed from the skin. Another option is to remove the fluid inside the bumps (termed curettage). Lasers also can remove molluscum bumps.

All three options may be a little painful and should only be done by a health care professional. Both curettage and cryotherapy methods may leave scars. In a small percentage of cases, natural healing of molluscum contagiosum bumps leads to scars regardless of type of therapy.

Once I am cured can I be reinfected with molluscum contagiosum?

Yes. Recovery from one infection with molluscum does not prevent future infections with molluscum so it is important not to pick at or scratch other people's skin.

Are there any complications of molluscum contagiosum infection?

The most common complication is a secondary infection caused by bacteria. Additionally, the removal of bumps by scratching, freezing (cryotherapy), or fluid removal (curettage) can leave scars on the skin.

What do I need to know about swimming pools and molluscum?

Some investigations report that spread of molluscum contagiosum is increased in swimming pools. However, it has not been proven how or under what circumstances swimming pools might increase spread of the virus. Activities related to swimming might be the cause. For example, the virus might spread from one person to another if they share a towel or toys. More research is needed to understand if and for how long the molluscum virus can live in swimming pool water and if such water can infect swimmers.

Open sores and breaks in the skin can become infected by many different germs. Therefore, people with open sores or breaks from any cause should not go into swimming pools.

If a person has molluscum bumps, the following recommendations should be followed when swimming:

- Cover all visible bumps with watertight bandages.

- Dispose of all used bandages at home.

- Do not share towels, kickboards or other equipment, or toys.

I have a weakened immune system. How could molluscum contagiosum affect me?

> **✔ Quick Tip**
>
> It is not a good idea to try to remove the molluscum growths or to get rid of the fluid inside them yourself. There are three important reasons not to treat the bumps without seeing a doctor first:
>
> - The treatment may be painful.
>
> - You might spread the bumps to another part of your body or to another person.
>
> - By scratching and scraping the skin you might cause a more serious bacterial infection.
>
> Be aware that some treatments available through the internet are not effective and may even be harmful.

Persons with weakened immune systems (such as cancer, organ transplantation, HIV etc.) are at increased risk for catching molluscum and may develop very large growths (the size of a dime or larger—at least 15 millimeters in diameter). Bumps may be anywhere on the body but tend to occur on the face and not to go away by themselves.

Treatment of molluscum is more difficult among persons with weakened immune systems. The best treatment is to strengthen the immune system by treating the primary problem.

The risk of a secondary infection caused by bacteria is always present. Your health care provider will discuss possible treatments for molluscum and ways to improve your overall health.

Since molluscum contagiosum virus is a poxvirus, does the smallpox vaccination protect me from getting molluscum contagiosum?

No, the smallpox vaccination will not protect you from becoming infected with molluscum contagiosum virus. Although both molluscum contagiosum virus and smallpox (variola) virus are from the same group of viruses (poxviruses), they have significantly different genetic makeup and are easily distinguished by your immune system.

Chapter 64

Human Immunodeficiency Virus (HIV) And Acquired Immune Deficiency Syndrome (AIDS)

What is HIV and how can I get it?

HIV—the human immunodeficiency virus—is a virus that kills your body's CD4 cells. CD4 cells (also called T-helper cells) help your body fight off infection and disease. HIV can be passed from person to person if someone with HIV infection has sex with or shares drug injection needles with another person. It also can be passed from a mother to her baby when she is pregnant, when she delivers the baby, or if she breastfeeds her baby.

What is AIDS?

AIDS—the acquired immunodeficiency syndrome—is a disease you get when HIV destroys your body's immune system. Normally, your immune system helps you fight off illness. When your immune system fails you can become very sick and can die.

About This Chapter: Information in this chapter is from "HIV and AIDS: Are You at Risk?" a publication of the Centers for Disease Control and Prevention, August 2007.

What do I need to know about HIV?

The first cases of AIDS were identified in the United States in 1981, but AIDS most likely existed here and in other parts of the world for many years before that time. In 1984 scientists proved that HIV causes AIDS.

Anyone can get HIV. The most important thing to know is how you can get the virus. These are ways you can get HIV:

- By having unprotected sex—sex without a condom—with someone who has HIV. The virus can be in an infected person's blood, semen, or vaginal secretions and can enter your body through tiny cuts or sores in your skin, or in the lining of your vagina, penis, rectum, or mouth.

- By sharing a needle and syringe to inject drugs or sharing drug equipment used to prepare drugs for injection with someone who has HIV.

- From a blood transfusion or blood clotting factor that you got before 1985. (But today it is unlikely you could get infected that way because all blood in the United States has been tested for HIV since 1985.)

These are ways you **cannot** get HIV:

- By working with or being around someone who has HIV

- From sweat, spit, tears, clothes, drinking fountains, phones, toilet seats, or through everyday things like sharing a meal

- From insect bites or stings

- From donating blood

- From a closed-mouth kiss (but there is a very small chance of getting it from open-mouthed or "French" kissing with an infected person because of possible blood contact)

> **✤ It's A Fact!!**
> Babies born to women with HIV also can become infected during pregnancy, birth, or breast-feeding.

How can I protect myself?

- **Don't share needles and syringes used to inject drugs, steroids, vitamins, or for tattooing or body piercing.** Also, don't share equipment ("works") used to prepare drugs to be injected. Many people have been infected with HIV, hepatitis, and other germs this way. Germs from an infected person can stay in a needle and then be injected directly into the next person who uses the needle.

- **The surest way to avoid transmission of sexually transmitted diseases (STDs) is to abstain from sexual intercourse, or to be in a long-term mutually monogamous relationship with a partner who has been tested and you know is uninfected.**

- **For persons whose sexual behaviors place them at risk for STDs, correct and consistent use of the male latex condom can reduce the risk of STD transmission.** However, no protective method is 100 percent effective, and condom use cannot guarantee absolute protection against any STD. The more sex partners you have, the greater your chances are of getting HIV or other diseases passed through sex.

- **Condoms used with a lubricant are less likely to break. However, condoms with the spermicide nonoxynol-9 are not recommended for STD/HIV prevention.** Condoms must be used correctly and consistently to be effective and protective. Incorrect use can lead to condom slippage or breakage, thus diminishing the protective effect. Inconsistent use, e.g., failure to use condoms with every act of intercourse, can result in STD transmission because transmission can occur with a single act of intercourse.

- **Don't share razors or toothbrushes because they may have the blood of another person on them.**

- **If you are pregnant or think you might be soon, talk to a doctor or your local health department about being tested for HIV.** If you have HIV, drug treatments are available to help you and they can reduce the chance of passing HIV to your baby.

How do I know if I have HIV or AIDS?

You might have HIV and still feel perfectly healthy. The only way to know for sure if you are infected or not is to be tested. Talk with a knowledgeable health care provider or counselor both before and after you are tested. You can go to your doctor or health department for testing.

✔ Quick Tip
To find out where to go in your area for HIV counseling
and testing, call your local health department.

Your doctor or health care provider can give you a confidential HIV test. The information on your HIV test and test results are confidential, as is your other medical information. This means it can be shared only with people authorized to see your medical records. You can ask your doctor, health care provider, or HIV counselor at the place you are tested to explain who can obtain this information. For example, you may want to ask whether your insurance company could find out your HIV status if you make a claim for health insurance benefits or apply for life insurance or disability insurance.

The Centers for Disease Control and Prevention (CDC) recommends that everyone know their HIV status. How often you should have an HIV test depends on your circumstances. If you have never been tested for HIV, you should be tested. CDC recommends being tested at least once a year if you do things, such as the following, that can transmit HIV infection:

- Injecting drugs or steroids with used injection equipment
- Having sex for money or drugs
- Having sex with an HIV-infected person
- Having more than one sex partner since your HIV test
- Having a sex partner who has had other sex partners since your last HIV test

In many states, you can be tested anonymously. These tests are usually given at special places known as anonymous testing sites. When you get an anonymous HIV test, the testing site records only a number or code with the test result, not your name. A counselor gives you this number at the time your blood, saliva, or urine is taken for the test, then you return to the testing site (or perhaps call the testing site, for example with home collection kits) and give them your number or code to learn the results of your test.

❖ **It's A Fact!!**

You are more likely to test positive for (be infected with) HIV if these statements apply you:

- Have ever shared injection drug needles and syringes or "works"

- Have ever had sex without a condom with someone who had HIV

- Have ever had a sexually transmitted disease, like chlamydia or gonorrhea

- Received a blood transfusion or a blood clotting factor between 1978 and 1985

- Have ever had sex with someone who has done any of those things

If you have been tested for HIV and the result is negative and you never do things that might transmit HIV infection, then you and your health care provider can decide whether you need to get tested again.

What can I do if the test shows I have HIV?

Although HIV is a very serious infection, many people with HIV and AIDS are living longer, healthier lives today, thanks to new and effective treatments. It is very important to make sure you have a doctor who knows how to treat HIV. If you don't know which doctor to use, talk with a health care professional or trained HIV counselor. If you are pregnant or are planning to become pregnant, this is especially important.

There also are other things you can do for yourself to stay healthy. Here are a few:

- **Follow your doctor's instructions.** Keep your appointments. Your doctor may prescribe medicine for you. Take the medicine just the way he or she tells you to because taking only some of your medicine gives your HIV infection more chance to grow.

- **Get immunizations (shots) to prevent infections such as pneumonia and flu.** Your doctor will tell you when to get these shots.

- **If you smoke or if you use drugs not prescribed by your doctor, quit.**

- **Eat healthy foods.** This will help keep you strong, keep your energy and weight up, and help your body protect itself.

- **Exercise regularly to stay strong and fit.**

- **Get enough sleep and rest.**

Chapter 65

Young People
And HIV

Young people in the United States continue to be at risk for human immunodeficiency virus (HIV) and acquired immune deficiency syndrome (AIDS). At the end of 2007, in 47 states, the District of Columbia, and five U.S. dependent areas with confidential name-based HIV infection surveillance, 54,108 young people ages 13–24 were living with HIV, comprising 16 percent of persons aged 13–24 at diagnosis.[1] But experts believe young people may suffer from up to 30 percent of all cases of HIV in the United States.[2] Youth of color and young men who have sex with men continue to be most at risk. It is important to promote programs that help young people lessen risky sexual behaviors by encouraging condom use, delay in sexual initiation, partner reduction, and early HIV testing and treatment. But research has shown that even when risk factors are equal, minority youth are more at risk for HIV. As such it is essential that research and resources be directed toward addressing the underlying social forces that contribute to these disparities and that policies and programs promote structural and social changes to ameliorate these factors.

HIV Among Young People 13–24 In The United States: Racial And Sexual Minority Youth Are At Greatly Disproportionate Risk

- From 2004–2007, 72 percent of HIV/AIDS diagnoses in young people aged 13–24 were in males, and 28 percent were in females. The majority of HIV/AIDS cases diagnosed among young men were attributed to male-to-male sexual contact. High-risk heterosexual contact attributed to the majority of HIV/AIDS cases diagnosed among young women.[3]

- In 2007, African Americans/blacks and Latinos/Hispanics accounted for 87 percent of all new HIV infections among 13- to 19-year-olds and 79 percent of HIV infections among 20- to 24-year-olds in the United States even though, together, they represent only about 32 percent of people these ages. Asian and Pacific Islanders (APIs) and American Indians and Alaska Natives account for about one percent of new HIV infections among young people ages 13–24.

- Young women of color suffer disproportionate rates—in 2007, African American/black and Latina/Hispanic women accounted for 82 percent of new infections in 13- to 24-year-old women in the United States, even though, together, they represent only about 26 percent of U.S. women these ages. In addition, African American/black women account for 62 percent and Latinas for 19 percent of cumulative AIDS cases among women ages 13–24.[4]

- Most young men who have HIV acquired it through male-to-male sexual contact, and the risk is increasing for young men who have sex with men (MSM). Between 2004 and 2007, HIV/AIDS cases among young men ages 13–24 who have sex with men increased across all ethnic groups, with young African American/black men most greatly affected.[5]

    - From 2004–2007, 87 percent of HIV/AIDS cases among young men ages 13–19 and 83 percent of HIV/AIDS cases among young men ages 20–24 were attributed to male-to-male sexual contact.[3]

- Sixty-two percent of HIV/AIDS infections among young men who have sex with men were in African Americans/blacks; 17 percent in Latinos/Hispanics; and 19 percent in whites.[5]

- From 2001–2005, cases of HIV/AIDS among young African American/black men ages 13–24 who have sex with men increased by 70 percent.[5]

Sexual Risk Behaviors Put Many Young People In Danger

- From 1991–2009, the percentage of high school students reporting that they had ever had sexual intercourse decreased from 54.1 percent to 46 percent. In 2009, 24.0 percent of Asian, 42.0 percent of white, 47.9 percent of Native Hawaiian or other Pacific Islander, 49.1 percent of Latino/Hispanic, 59.4 percent of American Indian/Alaskan Native, and 65.2 percent of black students reported that they had ever had sexual intercourse.[6]

- In 2009, the percentage of high school students reporting that they had sexual intercourse with four or more people during their life was highest among black students (28.6 percent) and American Indian/Alaskan Native students (23.4 percent). Eighteen percent (18.4 percent) of Native Hawaiian or other Pacific Islander, 14.2 percent of Latino/Hispanic students, 10.5 percent of white students, and 5.2 percent of Asian students reported having four or more partners.[6]

- Among sexually active high school students in 2009, 61.1 percent reported using a condom at most recent sex. Male students were significantly more likely to report condom use than female students (68.6 percent versus 53.9 percent, respectively). The prevalence of having used a condom during most recent sex was higher among white students (63.3 percent) and black students (62.4 percent) than Latino/Hispanic students (54.9 percent).[6]

- Research has shown that many young people are not concerned about becoming infected with HIV.[7,8] In addition, young people experience many barriers to HIV testing and are more likely than other population groups to not get tested for HIV.[9,10]

- In addition, many young people are unaware of their HIV status. Nationwide, only 13 percent of high school students have been tested for HIV. The prevalence of HIV testing was higher among black high school students (22 percent) than Latino/Hispanic (13 percent) and white (11 percent) students.[11] In 2006, 16 percent of young adults 18–24 reported that they had been tested for HIV in the past 12 months.[12] A study in six major cities found that among 15- to 22-year-old MSM in the United States, about three-quarters of those testing positive for HIV were unaware they had the virus, and black MSM had nearly seven times greater odds of having unrecognized HIV infection as white men.[13]

- Concurrent partnerships (multiple simultaneous sexual relationships or sexual relationships that overlap in time) put many young people at greater risk for HIV infection.[14]

Factors Which Contribute To Unequal Risk For HIV/ AIDS

- Increasingly, scientists recognize sexual networks, or connections between people living in the same community, as a driving force behind the HIV epidemic, especially for African Americans. Young people living in communities with high HIV prevalence are more at risk for HIV even if risk behaviors are the same as young people living in a community with lower HIV prevalence.[15, 16, 17, 18]

- Dating violence and sexual assault play a role in HIV transmission. Twenty percent of youth report experiencing dating violence. Women who experience dating violence are less likely to use condoms and feel more uncomfortable negotiating condom use. In one study, half of girls who reported HIV or sexually transmitted infections (STIs) had been physically or sexually abused.[19, 20, 21, 22]

- A study among black women in the South, a region with unusually high rates of HIV, concluded that socioeconomic factors, including financial dependence on male partners, feeling invincible, and low self-esteem, place young black women at risk for HIV/AIDS.[23]

- Having an STI (sexually transmitted infection) puts youth more at risk for HIV.[24] Almost half of the U.S.'s over 19 million STI infections each year occur in youth ages 15–24.[25] A recent study found that one in four young women ages 15–19 has an STI.[26] Young people of color experience STIs in greater numbers than White youth—African American and Hispanic Latino youth constituted 68 percent of Chlamydia cases among young people ages 15–24 and 82 percent of gonorrhea cases among young people ages 15–24 even though they make up only 30 percent of the population.[27]

Effective Strategies For HIV Prevention Among Young People

No single strategy will work to reduce HIV/AIDS infection among young people. However, research has shown that culturally competent, honest programs, that include information about abstinence, contraception, and condoms, can be effective in helping youth reduce risk behaviors.[28,29] In addition, open and honest parent-child communication about HIV and its prevention can aid youth in making good decisions.[30,31] Finally, resources must be directed at understanding the epidemic's impact on youth; at remedying the socioeconomic disparities which contribute to the epidemic; and at developing and testing a vaccine.

References

1. HIV/AIDS Surveillance: General Epidemiology (Through 2007). Centers for Disease Control and Prevention, 2009. Accessed from http://www.cdc.gov/hiv/topics/surveillance/resources/slides/general/slides/general.pdf on 3/22/10.

2. Morris, M., Handcock, M.S., Miller W.C., Ford, C.A. Schmitz, J.L., Hobbs, M.M., Cohen, M.S., Harris K.M., Udry J.R. Prevalence of HIV Infection Among Young Adults in the United States: Results from the Add Health Study. *American Journal of Public Health*. 2006 June: 96(6): 1091–1097.

3. HIV/AIDS Surveillance in Adolescents and Young Adults (Through 2007). Centers for Disease Control and Prevention, 2009. Accessed from http://www.cdc.gov/hiv/topics/surveillance/resources/slides/adolescents/slides/Adolescents.pdf on 3/22/10.

4. Cases of HIV Infection and AIDS in the United States and Dependent Areas, by Race/Ethnicity, 2003–2007. *HIV/AIDS Surveillance Supplemental Report, 2009*: 14(No.2). Accessed from http://www.cdc.gov/hiv/topics/surveillance/resources/reports/2009supp_vol14no2/pdf/HIVAIDS_SSR_Vol14_No2.pdf.

5. HIV/AIDS Surveillance in Men who have Sex with Men. Centers for Disease Control and Prevention, 2009. Accessed from http://www.cdc.gov/hiv/topics/surveillance/resources/slides/msm/slides/msm.pdf on 3/22/2010.

6. Centers for Disease Control and Prevention. Youth risk behavior surveillance system, United States 2009. *Morbidity and Mortality Weekly Report 2010*: 57(SS–5): 1–148.

7. Kaiser Family Foundation. National Survey of Teens on HIV/AIDS, 2000.

8. O'Sullivan L.F., Udell, W., Patel V.L. Young urban adults' heterosexual risk encounters and perceived risk and safety: a structured diary study. *Journal of Sex Research 2006*; 43(4):343–351.

9. Henry-Reid, L.M., Rodriquez F, Bell, M.A. et al. Youth counseled for HIV testing in school-and hospital-based clinics. *JAMA 1998*; 90:287–92.

10. Peralta, L., Deeds, B.G., Hipszer, S., Ghalib, K. Barriers and facilitators to adolescent HIV testing. *AIDS Patient Care STDS. 2007*; 21(6) 400–408.

11. Centers for Disease Control and Prevention. HIV testing among high school students—United States, 2007. *Morbidity and Mortality Weekly Report June 2009*: 58(24) 665–668.

12. Centers for Disease Control and Prevention. Persons Tested for HIV—United States, 2006. *Morbidity and Mortality Weekly Report August 8, 2008*: 57(31); 845–849.

13. MacKellar, D. et al, Unrecognized HIV infection, risk behaviors, and perception of risk among young men who have sex with men: opportunities for advancing HIV prevention in the third decade of HIV/AIDS. *Journal of AIDS*, Vol.38, No.5, 2005.

14. Gorback, P.M., Drumright L.N., Holmes K.K., Discord, discordance, and concurrency: comparing individual and partnership-level analyses of new

partnerships of young adults at risk of sexually transmitted infections. *Sexual Transmitted Diseases*. 2005 January; 32(1):7–12.

15. Millett et al. Explaining disparities in HIV infection among black and white men who have sex with men: a meta-analysis of HIV risk behaviors. *AIDS 21* (15) 2083–2091.

16. Adimora et al. HIV and African Americans in the Southern United States: Sexual Networks and Social Context. *Sexually Transmitted Diseases 2006*: 33 (7 suppl): S39–45.

17. Hallfors DD et al. "Sexual and drug behavior patterns and HIV and STD racial disparities: the need for new directions." *American Journal of Public Health 2007*; 97(1): 125–132.

18. Adimora AA et al. Ending the epidemic of heterosexual HIV transmission among African Americans. *American Journal of Preventative Medicine 2009*: 37(5):468–471.

19. Roberts TA, Klein J. Intimate Partner Abuse and High-Risk Behavior in Adolescents. *Archives of Pediatrics & Adolescent Medicine 2003*; 157:375–380.

20. Silverman JG, Raj A, Clements K. Dating Violence and Associated Sexual Risk and Pregnancy Among Adolescent Girls in the United States. *Pediatrics 2004*;114(2):e220–e225.

21. Decker et al. Dating Violence and Sexually Transmitted Disease/HIV Testing and Diagnosis Among Adolescent Females. *Pediatrics 2005*; 116 (2): e272–276.

22. Raiford, J.L. et al. Effects of fear of abuse and possible STI acquisition on the sexual behavior of young African American women. *American Journal of Public Health 2009*; 99(6): 1067–1071.

23. CDC. HIV Transmission among Black Women—North Carolina, 2004. *MMWR* 2005; 54(4); 89–92.

24. The Role of STD Detection and Treatment in HIV Prevention—CDC Fact Sheet, Centers for Disease Control and Prevention. Accessed from http://www.cdc.gov/std/HIV/STDFact-STD&HIV.htm on 4/1/08.

25. Weinstock, H., et al. Sexually transmitted diseases among American youth: incidence and prevalence estimates, 2000. *Perspectives on Sexual and Reproductive Health 2004*;36(1):6–10.

26. Centers for Disease Control and Prevention. Oral Abstract D4a— Prevalence of Sexually Transmitted Infections and Bacterial Vaginosis among Female Adolescents in the United States: Data from the National Health and Nutritional Examination Survey (NHANES) 2003–2004. 2008 National STD Prevention Conference. Accessed from http://www .cdc.gov/stdconference/.

27. Centers for Disease Control and Prevention. *Sexually Transmitted Disease Surveillance, 2008*. Atlanta, GA: U.S. Department of Health and Human Services; November 2009.

28. Kirby D. *Emerging Answers: Research Findings on Programs to Reduce Teen Pregnancy and Sexually Transmitted Infections*. Washington, DC: National Campaign to Prevent Teen Pregnancy, 2007.

29. Alford S. *Science and Success, Second Edition: Sex Education and Other Programs that Work to Prevent Teen Pregnancy, HIV & Sexually Transmitted Infections*. Washington, DC: Advocates for Youth, 2008.

30. Resnick MD et al. Protecting adolescents from harm: findings from the national longitudinal study on adolescent health. *JAMA 1997*; 278:823–32.

31. Miller KS et al. Patterns of condom use among adolescents: the impact of mother-adolescent communication. *Am J Public Health 1998*; 88:1542–44.

Chapter 66

HIV Testing Among Adolescents

Making human immunodeficiency virus (HIV) testing a routine part of health care for adolescents and adults aged 13–64 years is one of the most important strategies recommended by the Centers for Disease Control and Prevention (CDC) for reducing the spread of HIV. State, local, and territorial education agencies are essential partners in this effort.

Why HIV Testing Is Important

- Of the more than 1 million persons in the United States living with HIV/acquired immune deficiency syndrome (AIDS), an estimated 21% are unaware they are infected. This percentage is even higher among certain populations: more than 50% of HIV-infected adolescents and, according to one study, nearly 80% of young HIV-infected men who have sex with men do not know their infection status.

- Early identification of HIV infection enables people to start treatment sooner, leading to better health outcomes and longer lives.

- Increasing the number of HIV-infected people who are aware of their status is an integral part of prevention. Studies show that people who know they are infected are far less likely to have unprotected sex than those who do not.

About This Chapter: Information in this chapter is from "HIV Testing Among Adolescents," a publication by the Centers for Disease Control and Prevention, February 2009.

- HIV testing presents a vital opportunity to teach—or remind—people how they can protect themselves and others from HIV/AIDS and other sexually transmitted diseases (STDs).

Why HIV Testing Is Important For Adolescents

Adolescents report multiple risk behaviors for HIV infection, including early sexual activity. Studies have revealed these statistics among U.S. high school students:

- Forty-eight percent have had sexual intercourse at least once (including 33% of ninth grade students and 65% of 12th grade students).

- Seven percent had sexual intercourse for the first time before age 13.

- Fifteen percent have had four or more sex partners (including 9% of ninth grade students and 22% of 12th grade students).

- Thirty-eight percent of sexually active students did not use a condom the last time they had sex (including 31% of ninth grade students and 46% of 12th grade students).

♣ It's A Fact!!
Many young people are already infected with HIV, and the numbers are increasing.

- Two percent have injected illegal drugs at least once.

- By the end of 2006, an estimated 56,500 young people aged 13–24 were living with HIV infection or AIDS.

- Approximately 19,200 adolescents and young adults aged 13–29 were newly infected with HIV during 2006. This age group represented about 34% of all new HIV infections that year.

- Since 1985, more than 6,600 cases of AIDS among youth aged 13–19 have been reported.

- Certain subpopulations are disproportionately affected by HIV/AIDS, including young men who have sex with men, African Americans, and Hispanics.

Data On HIV Testing Among Adolescents

Available National Data

The national Youth Risk Behavior Survey (YRBS) provides data on the percentage of students in grades 9–12 who have been tested for HIV. According to the 2007 survey, 13% of 9th–12th grade students had ever been tested for HIV. Testing rates varied by sex (15% among female students, 11% among male students), race/ethnicity (22% among black students, 13% among Hispanic students, 11% among white students), and grade (9% among ninth graders, increasing to 19% among 12th graders).

The Need For State And Local Data

Although the national YRBS data are useful for characterizing HIV testing trends nationwide, state and local data are needed to examine local trends in testing behaviors, identify gaps in testing for certain populations, and determine whether young people at risk are being tested.

✤ It's A Fact!!

States and localities looking to characterize HIV testing trends in their areas can add an optional question to their Youth Risk Behavior Survey (YRBS) questionnaires:

Have you ever been tested for HIV, the virus that causes AIDS?

A. Yes   B. No   C. Not sure

Three states added the HIV testing question to their YRBS in 2007: Connecticut, Massachusetts, and New Jersey. Both of the states with weighted data, Connecticut and Massachusetts, found that 14% of 9th–12th grade students had been tested for HIV. In these same two states, however, 37% and 39% of students, respectively, who had had sexual intercourse within the preceding three months had not used a condom the last time they had sex. These findings indicate a gap between engaging in risky behavior and being tested for HIV. Adding the HIV testing question to the YRBS can help states and districts identify such gaps, discover racial/ethnic disparities in testing, and prioritize interventions accordingly.

What Schools Are Doing To Support HIV Testing

The 2006 School Health Policies and Programs Study indicated that many U.S. high schools have already demonstrated their commitment to HIV education, counseling, and testing:

- Eighty-five percent teach, as part of required courses, how HIV is transmitted.

- Seventy-seven percent teach how HIV is diagnosed and treated.

- Seventy-six percent teach how to find valid information or services regarding HIV or HIV counseling or testing.

School health professionals are in an excellent position to identify and refer youth for HIV prevention, counseling, and testing services. A number of states, districts, and schools have taken an active role:

- Many schools maintain linkages with local health centers and community-based organizations to help students receive needed screenings and treatment.

- Some school-based health clinics offer HIV and other STD testing on site. For example, school-based health centers across Seattle provide free, on-site clinical services, including HIV and STD counseling and testing.

- In Philadelphia, all ninth grade and transfer students are offered STD testing at school, in collaboration with the health department. Students who test positive are provided STD treatment at school and referred locally for HIV testing.

- In Hawaii, Peer Education Program Coordinators are given sample HIV test kits to use when teaching school staff about HIV testing as part of World AIDS Day activities.

- In Puerto Rico, the Department of Health formed a cooperative agreement with the Department of Education to conduct HIV and STD counseling and testing in public high schools across the island.

Chapter 67

Pubic Lice ("Crabs")

What are pubic lice?

Also called crab lice or "crabs," pubic lice are parasitic insects found primarily in the pubic or genital area of humans. Pubic lice infestation is found worldwide and occurs in all races, ethnic groups, and levels of society.

What do pubic lice look like?

Pubic lice have forms: the egg (also called a nit), the nymph, and the adult.

Nit: Nits are lice eggs. They can be hard to see and are found firmly attached to the hair shaft. They are oval and usually yellow to white. Pubic lice nits take about 6–10 days to hatch.

Nymph: The nymph is an immature louse that hatches from the nit (egg). A nymph looks like an adult pubic louse but it is smaller. Pubic lice nymphs take about two to three weeks after hatching to mature into adults capable of reproducing. To live, a nymph must feed on blood.

Adult: The adult pubic louse resembles a miniature crab when viewed through a strong magnifying glass. Pubic lice have six legs; their two front legs are very large and look like the pincher claws of a crab. This is how they

About This Chapter: Information in this chapter is from "Pubic 'Crab' Lice: Frequently Asked Questions," and "Pubic 'Crab' Lice: Treatment," both fact sheets from the Centers for Disease Control and Prevention, November 2010.

got the nickname "crabs." Pubic lice are tan to grayish-white in color. Females lay nits and are usually larger than males. To live, lice must feed on blood. If the louse falls off a person, it dies within one to two days.

Where are pubic lice found?

Pubic lice usually are found in the genital area on pubic hair but they may occasionally be found on other coarse body hair, such as hair on the legs, armpits, mustache, beard, eyebrows, or eyelashes. Pubic lice on the eyebrows or eyelashes of children may be a sign of sexual exposure or abuse. Lice found on the head generally are head lice, not pubic lice.

What are the signs and symptoms of pubic lice?

Signs and symptoms of pubic lice include itching in the genital area and visible nits (lice eggs) or crawling lice.

> ♣ **It's A Fact!!**
> Animals do not get or spread pubic lice.
>
> Source: "FAQ," Centers for Disease Control and Prevention, 2010.

How did I get pubic lice?

Pubic lice usually are spread through sexual contact and are most common in adults. Pubic lice found on children may be a sign of sexual exposure or abuse. Occasionally, pubic lice may be spread by close personal contact or contact with articles such as clothing, bed linens, or towels that have been used by an infested person.

A common misconception is that pubic lice are spread easily by sitting on a toilet seat. This would be extremely rare because lice cannot live long away from a warm human body, and they do not have feet designed to hold onto or walk on smooth surfaces such as toilet seats.

Persons infested with pubic lice should be investigated for the presence of other sexually transmitted diseases (STDs).

How is a pubic lice infestation diagnosed?

A pubic lice infestation is diagnosed by finding a "crab" louse or egg (nit) on hair in the pubic region or, less commonly, elsewhere on the body (eyebrows, eyelashes, beard, mustache, armpit, perianal area, groin, trunk, scalp). Pubic

> ## ✤ It's A Fact!!
>
> Although pubic lice and nits can be large enough to be seen with the naked eye, a magnifying lens may be necessary to find lice or eggs.
>
> Source: "FAQ," Centers for Disease Control and Prevention, 2010.

lice may be difficult to find because there may be only a few. Pubic lice often attach themselves to more than one hair and generally do not crawl as quickly as head and body lice. If crawling lice are not seen, finding nits in the pubic area strongly suggests that a person is infested and should be treated. If you are unsure about infestation or if treatment is not successful, see a health care provider for a diagnosis.

How is a pubic lice infestation treated?

A lice-killing lotion containing 1% permethrin or a mousse containing pyrethrins and piperonyl butoxide can be used to treat pubic ("crab") lice. These products are available over-the-counter without a prescription at a local drug store or pharmacy. These medications are safe and effective when used exactly according to the instructions in the package or on the label.

Lindane shampoo is a prescription medication that can kill lice and lice eggs. However, lindane is not recommended as a first-line therapy. Lindane can be toxic to the brain and other parts of the nervous system; its use should be restricted to patients who have failed treatment with or cannot tolerate other medications that pose less risk. Lindane should not be used to treat premature infants, persons with a seizure disorder, women who are pregnant or breastfeeding, persons who have very irritated skin or sores where the lindane will be applied, infants, children, the elderly, and persons who weigh less than 110 pounds.

Malathion lotion 0.5% (Ovide) is a prescription medication that can kill lice and some lice eggs; however, malathion lotion (Ovide) currently has not been approved by the U.S. Food and Drug Administration (FDA) for treatment of pubic ("crab") lice.

Ivermectin has been used successfully to treat lice; however, ivermectin currently has not been approved by the FDA for treatment of lice.

How to treat pubic lice infestations:

Warning: See special instructions for treatment of lice and nits on eyebrows or eyelashes. The lice medications described in this section should not be used near the eyes.

1. Wash the infested area; towel dry.

2. Carefully follow the instructions in the package or on the label. Thoroughly saturate the pubic hair and other infested areas with lice medication. Leave medication on hair for the time recommended in the instructions. After waiting the recommended time, remove the medication by following carefully the instructions on the label or in the box.

3. Following treatment, most nits will still be attached to hair shafts. Nits may be removed with fingernails or by using a fine-toothed comb.

4. Put on clean underwear and clothing after treatment.

5. To kill any lice or nits remaining on clothing, towels, or bedding, machine wash and machine dry those items that the infested person used during the two to three days before treatment. Use hot water (at least 130°F) and the hot dryer cycle.

6. Items that cannot be laundered can be dry-cleaned or stored in a sealed plastic bag for two weeks.

7. All sex partners from within the previous month should be informed that they are at risk for infestation and should be treated.

8. Persons should avoid sexual contact with their sex partner(s) until both they and their partners have been successfully treated and reevaluated to rule out persistent infestation.

9. Repeat treatment in 9–10 days if live lice are still found.

10. Persons with pubic lice should be evaluated for other STDs.

Special instructions for treatment of lice and nits found on eyebrows or eyelashes:

- If only a few live lice and nits are present, it may be possible to remove these with fingernails or a nit comb.

- If additional treatment is needed for lice or nits on the eyelashes, careful application of ophthalmic-grade petrolatum ointment (only available by prescription) to the eyelid margins two to four times a day for 10 days is effective. Regular petrolatum (e.g., Vaseline) should not be used because it can irritate the eyes if applied.

☞ Remember!!

This information is not meant to be used for self-diagnosis or as a substitute for consultation with a health care provider. If you have any questions about the disease described above or think that you may have a parasitic infection, consult a health care provider.

Source: "Treatment," Centers for Disease
Control and Prevention, 2010.

Chapter 68

Trichomoniasis

What is trichomoniasis?

Trichomoniasis is a common sexually transmitted disease (STD) that affects both women and men, although symptoms are more common in women.

How common is trichomoniasis?

Trichomoniasis is the most common curable STD in young, sexually active women. An estimated 7.4 million new cases occur each year in women and men.

How do people get trichomoniasis?

Trichomoniasis is caused by the single-celled protozoan parasite, *Trichomonas vaginalis*. The vagina is the most common site of infection in women, and the urethra (urine canal) is the most common site of infection in men.

The parasite is sexually transmitted through penis-to-vagina intercourse or vulva-to-vulva (the genital area outside the vagina) contact with an infected partner. Women can acquire the disease from infected men or women, but men usually contract it only from infected women.

About This Chapter: Information in this chapter is from "Trichomoniasis," a fact sheet from the Centers for Disease Control and Prevention, December 2007.

What are the signs and symptoms?

Most men with trichomoniasis do not have signs or symptoms; however, some men may temporarily have an irritation inside the penis, mild discharge, or slight burning after urination or ejaculation.

Some women have signs or symptoms of infection which include a frothy, yellow-green vaginal discharge with a strong odor. The infection also may cause discomfort during intercourse and urination, as well as irritation and itching of the female genital area. In rare cases, lower abdominal pain can occur. Symptoms usually appear in women within five to 28 days of exposure.

What are the complications of trichomoniasis?

The genital inflammation caused by trichomoniasis can increase a woman's susceptibility to human immunodeficiency virus (HIV) infection if she is exposed to the virus. Having trichomoniasis may increase the chance that an HIV-infected woman passes HIV to her sex partner(s).

How does trichomoniasis affect a pregnant woman and her baby?

Pregnant women with trichomoniasis may have babies who are born early or with low birth weight (low birth weight is less than 5.5 pounds).

How is trichomoniasis diagnosed?

For both men and women, a health care provider must perform a physical examination and laboratory test to diagnose trichomoniasis. The parasite is harder to detect in men than in women.

❖ It's A Fact!!
In women infected with trichomoniasis, a pelvic examination can reveal small red ulcerations (sores) on the vaginal wall or cervix.

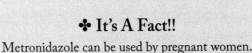

❖ It's A Fact!!
Metronidazole can be used by pregnant women.

What is the treatment for trichomoniasis?

Trichomoniasis can usually be cured with prescription drugs, either metronidazole or tinidazole, given by mouth in a single dose. The symptoms of trichomoniasis in infected men may disappear within a few weeks without treatment. However, an infected man, even a man who has never had symptoms or whose symptoms have stopped, can continue to infect or reinfect a female partner until he has been treated. Therefore, both partners should be treated at the same time to eliminate the parasite. Persons being treated for trichomoniasis should avoid sex until they and their sex partners complete treatment and have no symptoms.

Having trichomoniasis once does not protect a person from getting it again. Following successful treatment, people can still be susceptible to reinfection.

How can trichomoniasis be prevented?

The surest way to avoid transmission of sexually transmitted diseases is to abstain from sexual contact, or to be in a long-term mutually monogamous relationship with a partner who has been tested and is known to be uninfected.

Latex male condoms, when used consistently and correctly, can reduce the risk of transmission of trichomoniasis.

Any genital symptom such as discharge or burning during urination or an unusual sore or rash should be a signal to stop having sex and to consult a health care provider immediately. A person diagnosed with trichomoniasis (or any other STD) should receive treatment and should notify all recent sex partners so that they can see a health care provider and be treated. This reduces the risk that the sex partners will develop complications from trichomoniasis and reduces the risk that the person with trichomoniasis will become rein-fected. Sex should be stopped until the person with trichomoniasis and all of his or her recent partners complete treatment for trichomoniasis and have no symptoms.

Chapter 69

Scabies

What is scabies?

Scabies is an infestation of the skin by the human itch mite (*Sarcoptes scabiei var. hominis*). The microscopic scabies mite burrows into the upper layer of the skin where it lives and lays its eggs. The most common symptoms of scabies are intense itching and a pimple-like skin rash. The scabies mite usually is spread by direct, prolonged, skin-to-skin contact with a person who has scabies.

Scabies is found worldwide and affects people of all races and social classes. Scabies can spread rapidly under crowded conditions where close body and skin contact is frequent. Institutions such as nursing homes, extended-care facilities, and prisons are often sites of scabies outbreaks. Childcare facilities also are a common site of scabies infestations.

What is crusted (Norwegian) scabies?

Crusted scabies is a severe form of scabies that can occur in some persons who are immunocompromised (have a weak immune system), elderly, disabled, or debilitated. It is also called Norwegian scabies. Persons with crusted scabies have thick crusts of skin that contain large numbers of scabies mites and eggs. Persons with crusted scabies are very contagious to other persons

About This Chapter: Information in this chapter is from "Scabies Frequently Asked Questions (FAQs)," a fact sheet from the Centers for Disease Control and Prevention, November 2010.

and can spread the infestation easily both by direct skin-to-skin contact and by contamination of items such as their clothing, bedding, and furniture. Persons with crusted scabies may not show the usual signs and symptoms of scabies such as the characteristic rash or itching (pruritus). Persons with crusted scabies should receive quick and aggressive medical treatment for their infestation to prevent outbreaks of scabies.

How soon after infestation do symptoms of scabies begin?

If a person has never had scabies before, symptoms may take as long as four to six weeks to begin. It is important to remember that an infested person can spread scabies during this time, even if he/she does not have symptoms yet.

In a person who has had scabies before, symptoms usually appear much sooner (one to four days) after exposure.

What are the signs and symptoms of scabies infestation?

The most common signs and symptoms of scabies are intense itching (pruritus), especially at night, and a pimple-like (papular) itchy rash. The itching and rash each may affect much of the body or be limited to common sites such as the wrist, elbow, armpit, webbing between the fingers, nipple, penis, waist, beltline, and buttocks. The rash also can include tiny blisters (vesicles) and scales. Scratching the rash can cause skin sores; sometimes these sores become infected by bacteria.

Tiny burrows sometimes are seen on the skin; these are caused by the female scabies mite tunneling just beneath the surface of the skin. These burrows appear as tiny raised and crooked (serpiginous) grayish-white or skin-colored lines on the skin surface. Because mites are often few in number (only 10–15 mites per person), these burrows may be difficult to find. They are found most often in the webbing between the fingers, in the skin folds on the wrist, elbow, or knee, and on the penis, breast, or shoulder blades.

♣ It's A Fact!!

The head, face, neck, palms, and soles often are involved in scabies infections of infants and very young children, but usually not adults and older children.

Persons with crusted (Norwegian) scabies may not show the usual signs and symptoms of scabies such as the characteristic rash or itching (pruritus).

How did I get scabies?

Scabies usually is spread by direct, prolonged, skin-to-skin contact with a person who has scabies. Contact generally must be prolonged; a quick handshake or hug usually will not spread scabies. Scabies is spread easily to sexual partners and household members. Scabies in adults frequently is sexually acquired.

Scabies sometimes is spread indirectly by sharing articles such as clothing, towels, or bedding used by an infested person; however, such indirect spread can occur much more easily when the infested person has crusted scabies.

How is scabies infestation diagnosed?

Diagnosis of a scabies infestation usually is made based on the customary appearance and distribution of the rash and the presence of burrows. Whenever possible, the diagnosis of scabies should be confirmed by identifying the mite, mite eggs, or mite fecal matter (scybala). This can be done by carefully removing a mite from the end of its burrow using the tip of a needle or by obtaining skin scraping to examine under a microscope for mites, eggs, or mite fecal matter. It is important to remember that a person can still be infested even if mites, eggs, or fecal matter cannot be found; typically fewer than 10–15 mites can be present on the entire body of an infested person who is otherwise healthy. However, persons with crusted scabies can be infested with thousands of mites and should be considered highly contagious.

How long can scabies mites live?

On a person, scabies mites can live for as long as one to two months. Off a person, scabies mites usually do not survive more than 48–72 hours. Scabies mites will die if exposed to a temperature of 50° C (122° F) for 10 minutes.

Can scabies be treated?

Yes. Products used to treat scabies are called scabicides because they kill scabies mites; some also kill eggs. Scabicides to treat human scabies are available only with a doctor's prescription; no over-the-counter (nonprescription) products have been tested and approved for humans.

Always follow carefully the instructions provided by the doctor and pharmacist, as well as those contained in the box or printed on the label. When treating adults and older children, scabicide cream or lotion is applied to all areas of the body from the neck down to the feet and toes; when treating infants and young children, the cream or lotion also is applied to the head and neck. The medication should be left on the body for the recommended time before it is washed off. Clean clothes should be worn after treatment.

In addition to the infested person, treatment also is recommended for household members and sexual contacts, particularly those who have had prolonged skin-to-skin contact with the infested person. All persons should be treated at the same time in order to prevent reinfestation. Retreatment may be necessary if itching continues more than two to four weeks after treatment or if new burrows or rash continue to appear.

Who should be treated for scabies?

Anyone who is diagnosed with scabies, as well as his or her sexual partners and other contacts who have had prolonged skin-to-skin contact with the infested person, should be treated. Treatment is recommended for members of the same household as the person with scabies, particularly those persons who have had prolonged skin-to-skin contact with the infested person. All persons should be treated at the same time to prevent reinfestation.

> ✔ **Quick Tip**
> Never use a scabicide intended for veterinary or agricultural use to treat humans.

How soon after treatment will I feel better?

If itching continues more than two to four weeks after initial treatment or if new burrows or rash continue to appear (if initial treatment includes more than one application or dose, then the two to four week time period begins after the last application or dose), retreatment with scabicide may be necessary; seek the advice of a physician.

> ♣ **It's A Fact!!**
> Retreatment of scabies may be necessary if itching continues more than two to four weeks after treatment or if new burrows or rash continue to appear.

Did I get scabies from my pet?

No. Animals do not spread human scabies. Pets can become infested with a different kind of scabies mite that does not survive or reproduce on humans but causes "mange" in animals. If an animal with "mange" has close contact with a person, the animal mite can get under the person's skin and cause temporary itching and skin irritation. However, the animal mite cannot reproduce on a person and will die on its own in a couple of days. Although the person does not need to be treated, the animal should be treated because its mites can continue to burrow into the person's skin and cause symptoms until the animal has been treated successfully.

Can scabies be spread by swimming in a public pool?

Scabies is very unlikely to be spread by water in a swimming pool. Except for a person with crusted scabies, only about 10–15 scabies mites are present on an infested person; it is extremely unlikely that any would emerge from under wet skin.

> ♣ **It's A Fact!!**
> Because persons with crusted scabies are considered very infectious, careful vacuuming of furniture and carpets in rooms used by these persons is recommended.

How can I remove scabies mites from my house or carpet?

Scabies mites do not survive more than two to three days away from human skin. Items such as bedding, clothing, and towels used by a person with scabies can be decontaminated by machine washing in hot water and drying using the hot cycle or by dry-cleaning. Items that cannot be washed or dry-cleaned can be decontaminated by removing from any body contact for at least 72 hours.

Fumigation of living areas is unnecessary.

My spouse and I were diagnosed with scabies. After several treatments, he/she still has symptoms while I am cured. Why?

The rash and itching of scabies can persist for several weeks to a month after treatment, even if the treatment was successful and all the mites and eggs have been killed. Your health care provider may prescribe additional medication to relieve itching if it is severe. Symptoms that persist for longer than two weeks after treatment can be due to a number of reasons.

If I come in contact with a person who has scabies, should I treat myself?

No. If a person thinks he or she might have scabies, he/she should contact a doctor. The doctor can examine the person, confirm the diagnosis of scabies, and prescribe an appropriate treatment. Products used to treat scabies in humans are available only with a doctor's prescription.

☞ Remember!!

Sleeping with or having sex with any scabies-infested person presents a high risk for transmission.

Chapter 70

STDs And Pregnancy

Can pregnant women become infected with sexually transmitted diseases (STDs)?

Yes, women who are pregnant can become infected with the same STDs as women who are not pregnant. Pregnancy does not provide women or their babies any protection against STDs. The consequences of an STD can be significantly more serious, even life threatening, for a woman and her baby if the woman becomes infected with an STD while pregnant. It is important that women be aware of the harmful effects of STDs and know how to protect themselves and their children against infection.

How common are STDs in pregnant women in the United States?

Some STDs, such as genital herpes and bacterial vaginosis, are quite common in pregnant women in the United States. Other STDs, notably human immunodeficiency virus (HIV) and syphilis, are much less common in pregnant women. Table 70.1 shows the estimated number of pregnant women in the United States who are infected with specific STDs each year.

About This Chapter: Information in this chapter is from "STDS & Pregnancy," a fact sheet from the Centers for Disease Control and Prevention, January 2008.

Table 70.1. STDs In U.S. Women

STDs	Estimated Number Of Pregnant Women
Bacterial vaginosis	1,080,000
Herpes simplex virus 2	880,000
Chlamydia	100,000
Trichomoniasis	124,000
Gonorrhea	13,200
Hepatitis B	16,000
HIV	6,400
Syphilis	<1,000

How do STDs affect a pregnant woman and her baby?

STDs can have many of the same consequences for pregnant women as for women who are not pregnant. STDs can cause cervical and other cancers, chronic hepatitis, pelvic inflammatory disease, infertility, and other complications. Many STDs in women are silent; that is, without signs or symptoms.

STDs can be passed from a pregnant woman to the baby before, during, or after the baby's birth. Some STDs (like syphilis) cross the placenta and infect the baby while it is in the uterus (womb). Other STDs (like gonorrhea, chlamydia, hepatitis B, and genital herpes) can be transmitted from the mother to the baby during delivery as the baby passes through the birth canal. HIV can cross the placenta during pregnancy, infect the baby during the birth process, and unlike most other STDs, can infect the baby through breastfeeding.

❖ It's A Fact!!
A pregnant woman with an STD may also have early onset of labor, premature rupture of the membranes surrounding the baby in the uterus, and uterine infection after delivery.

The harmful effects of STDs in babies may include stillbirth (a baby that is born dead), low birth weight (less than five pounds), conjunctivitis (eye infection), pneumonia, neonatal sepsis (infection in the baby's bloodstream), neurologic damage, blindness, deafness, acute hepatitis, meningitis, chronic liver disease, and cirrhosis. Most of these problems can be prevented if the mother receives routine prenatal care, which includes screening tests for STDs starting early in pregnancy and repeated close to delivery, if necessary. Other problems can be treated if the infection is found at birth.

Should pregnant women be tested for STDs?

Yes, STDs affect women of every socio-economic and educational level, age, race, ethnicity, and religion. The *CDC 2006 Guidelines for Treatment of Sexually Transmitted Diseases* recommend that pregnant women be screened on their first prenatal visit for STDs which may include the following:

- Chlamydia
- Gonorrhea
- Hepatitis B
- HIV
- Syphilis

> ❖ **It's A Fact!!**
>
> Pregnant women should ask their doctors about getting tested for STDs, since some doctors do not routinely perform these tests. New and increasingly accurate tests continue to become available. Even if a woman has been tested in the past, she should be tested again when she becomes pregnant.

In addition, some experts recommend that women who have had a premature delivery in the past be screened and treated for bacterial vaginosis at the first prenatal visit.

Can STDs be treated during pregnancy?

Chlamydia, gonorrhea, syphilis, trichomoniasis, and bacterial vaginosis can be treated and cured with antibiotics during pregnancy. There is no cure for viral STDs, such as genital herpes and HIV, but antiviral medication may be appropriate for pregnant women with herpes and definitely is for those with HIV. For women who have active genital herpes lesions at the time of delivery, a cesarean delivery (C-section) may be performed to protect the newborn against infection. C-section is also an option for some HIV-infected women. Women who test negative for hepatitis B may receive the hepatitis B vaccine during pregnancy.

How can pregnant women protect themselves against infection?

The surest way to avoid transmission of sexually transmitted diseases is to abstain from sexual contact, or to be in a long-term mutually monogamous relationship with a partner who has been tested and is known to be uninfected.

Latex condoms, when used consistently and correctly, are highly effective in preventing transmission of HIV, the virus that causes acquired immune deficiency syndrome (AIDS). Latex condoms, when used consistently and correctly, can reduce the risk of transmission of gonorrhea, chlamydia, and trichomoniasis. Correct and consistent use of latex condoms can reduce the risk of genital herpes, syphilis, and chancroid only when the infected area or site of potential exposure is protected by the condom. Correct and consistent use of latex condoms may reduce the risk for genital human papillomavirus (HPV) and associated diseases (e.g. warts and cervical cancer).

Part Seven

If You Need More Information

Chapter 71

Resources For Additional Information About Sexual Development And Sexually Transmitted Diseases

Adolescent AIDS Program
Children's Hospital at Montefiore
Medical Center
111 East 210th Street
Bronx, NY 10467
Phone: 718-882-0232
Fax: 718-882-0432
Website:
http://www.adolescentaids.org
E-mail: info@adolescentaids.org

Advocates For Youth
2000 M Street NW, Suite 750
Washington, DC 20036
Phone: 202-419-3420
Fax: 202-419-1448
Website:
http://www.advocatesforyouth.org

American Academy of Family Physicians
11400 Tomahawk Creek Parkway
Leawood, KS 66211-2672
Toll-Free: 800-274-2237
Phone: 913-906-6000
Website: http://www.aafp.org
E-mail: fp@aafp.org

American Academy of Pediatrics
141 Northwest Point Boulevard
Elk Grove Village, IL 60007-1098
Phone: 847-434-4000
Fax: 847-434-8000
Website: http://www.aap.org

American Board of Obstetrics and Gynecology
2915 Vine Street
Dallas, TX 75204
Phone: 214-871-1619
Fax: 214-871-1943
Website: http://www.abog.org
E-mail: info@abog.org

American College of Nurse-Midwives
8403 Colesville Road
Suite 1550
Silver Spring, MD 20910-6374
Phone: 240-485-1800
Fax: 240-485-1818

American College of Obstetricians and Gynecologists (ACOG)
409 12th Street SW
P.O. Box 96920
Washington, DC 20090-6920
Phone: 202-638-5577
Website: http://www.acog.org

American Pregnancy Association
1425 Greenway Drive
Suite 440
Irving, TX 75038
Phone: 972-550-0140
Fax: 972-550-0800
Website:
http://www.americanpregnancy.org
E-mail:
Questions@AmericanPregnancy.org

American Psychological Association
750 First Street, NE
Washington, DC 20002-4242
Toll-Free: 800-374-2721
Phone: 202-336-5500
TDD/TTY: 202-336-6123
Website: http://www.apa.org

American Social Health Association
P.O. Box 13827
Research Triangle Park, NC 27709
Phone: 919-361-8400
Fax: 919-361-8425
Website:
http://www.ashastd.org
Teen-oriented website:
http://www.iwannaknow.org

Association of Reproductive Health Professionals (ARHP)
1901 L Street, NW
Suite 300
Washington, DC 20036
Phone: 202-466-3825
Fax: 202-466-3826
Website: www.arhp.org

Breastcancer.org
7 East Lancaster Avenue
3rd Floor
Ardmore, PA 19003
Website:
http://www.breastcancer.org

Boys Town
14100 Crawford Street
Boys Town, NE 68010
Toll Free: 800-448-3000
Phone: 402-498-1300
Fax: 402-498-1348
Website: http://boystown.org

Center for Adolescent Health
Johns Hopkins Bloomberg
School of Public Health
615 North Wolfe Street
Room E4612
Baltimore, MD 21205
Phone: 410-614-3953
Website: http://www.jhsph.edu/
adolescenthealth

Center for Young Women's Health
333 Longwood Avenue,
5th Floor
Boston, MA 02115
Phone: 617-355-2994
Fax: 617-730-0186
Website:
http://www.youngwomenshealth.org

**Centers for Disease
Control and Prevention**
1600 Clifton Road
Atlanta, GA 30333
Toll-Free: 800-232-4636
Website: http://www.cdc.gov

**Childhelp National
Child Abuse Hotline**
Toll-Free: 1-800-4-A-CHILD
(1-800-422-4453)

The Cleveland Clinic
9500 Euclid Avenue
Cleveland, Ohio 44195
Toll-Free: 800-223-2273
TTY: 216-444-0261

Endometriosis Association
8585 North 76th Place
Milwaukee, WI 53223
Phone: 414-355-2200
Fax: 414-355-6065
Website:
http://www.endometriosisassn.org

Endometriosis Research Center
630 Ibis Drive
Delray Beach, FL 33444
Toll-Free: 800-239-7280
Phone: 561-274-7442
Fax: 561-274-0931
Website: http://www.endocenter.org
E-mail: askerc@aol.com

Alan Guttmacher Institute
125 Maiden Lane, 7th Floor
New York, NY 10038
Toll-Free: 800-355-0244
Phone: 212-248-1111
Fax: 212-248-1951
Website: http://www.guttmacher.org
E-mail: info@guttmacher.org

GLBT National Help Center
2261 Market Street, PMB #296
San Francisco, CA 94114
Toll-Free: 888-843-4564
(National Hotline)
Toll-Free: 800-246-7743
(Youth Hotline)
Website: http://www.glnh.org/
E-mail:
info@GLBTNationalHelpCenter.org

Hormone Foundation
8401 Connecticut Avenue
Suite 900
Chevy Chase, MD 20815-5817
Toll-Free: 800-HORMONE
Fax: 301-941-0259
Website: http://www.hormone.org
E-mail: hormone@endo-society.org

Henry J. Kaiser Family Foundation
2400 Sand Hill Road
Menlo Park, CA 94025
Phone: 650-854-9400
Fax: 650-854-4800
Website: http://www.kff.org

**National Campaign to Prevent
Teen and Unplanned Pregnancy**
1776 Massachusetts Avenue, NW
Suite 200
Washington, DC 20036
Phone: 202-478-8500
Fax: 202-478-8588
Website: http://www.thenational-
campaign.org

National Cancer Institute
NCI Public Inquires Office
6116 Executive Boulevard
Suite 300
Bethesda, MD 20892-8322
Toll-Free: 800-4-CANCER
(800-422-6237)
TTY: 800-332-8615
Website: http://www.cancer.gov

**National Cervical Cancer
Coalition (NCCC)**
6520 Platt Ave. #693
West Hills, CA 91307
Toll-Free: 800-685-5531
Phone: 818-992-4242
Fax: 818-992-4178
Website: http://www.nccc-online.org
E-mail: info@nccc-online.org

**National Family Planning and
Reproductive Health Association**
1627 K Street, NW, 12th Floor
Washington, DC 20005
Phone: 202-293-3114
Website: http://www.nfprha.org
E-mail: info@nfprha.org

**National Human Genome
Research Institute**
National Institutes of Health
Building 31, Room 4B09
31 Center Drive, MSC 2152
9000 Rockville Pike
Bethesda, MD 20892-2152
Phone: 301-402-0911
Fax: 301-402-2218

**National Institute of Allergy
and Infectious Diseases**
NIAID Office of Communications
and Public Liaison
6610 Rockledge Drive, MSC 6612
Bethesda, MD 20892-6612
Toll-Free: 866-284-4107
TDD: 800-877-8339
Fax: 301-402-3573
Website: http://www.niaid.nih.gov

**National Institute of Arthritis and
Musculoskeletal and Skin Diseases
(NIAMS)**
Information Clearinghouse
National Institutes of Health
1 AMS Circle
Bethesda, MD 20892-3675
Phone: 301-495-4484
Toll-Free: 877-22-NIAMS
(226-4267)
TTY: 301-565-2966
Fax: 301-718-6366
Website: http://www.niams.nih.gov
E-mail: NIAMSinfo@mail.nih.gov

**National Institute of Child
Health and Human Development
(NICHD)**
31 Center Drive, Bldg. 31
Room 2A32, MSC 2425
Bethesda, MD 20892-2425
Toll-Free: 800-370-2943
Fax: 866-760-5847
TTY: 888-320-6942
Website: http://www.nichd.nih.gov

National Kidney Foundation
30 East 33rd Street
New York, NY 10016
Toll-Free: 800-622-9010
Phone: 212-889-2210
Fax: 212-689-9261
Website: http://www.kidney.org
E-mail: info@kidney.org

**National Kidney and
Urologic Diseases Information
Clearinghouse**
3 Information Way
Bethesda, MD 20892-3580
Phone: 800-891-5390
TTY: 866-569-1162
Fax: 703-738-4929
Website: http://kidney.niddk.nih.gov
E-mail: nkudic@info.niddk.nih.gov

**National Prevention Information
Network**
P.O. Box 6003
Rockville, MD 20849-6003
Toll-Free: 800-458-5231
Fax: 888-282-7681
Website: http://cdcnpin.org
E-mail: info@cdcnpin.org

**National Research Center for
Women & Families**
1701 K St. NW, Suite 700
Washington, DC 20006
Phone: 202-223-4000
Fax: 202-223-4242
E-mail: info@breastimplantinfo.org

**National Teen Dating
Abuse Helpline**
Toll-Free: 866-331-9474
TTY: 866-331-8453

**National Women's Health
Information Center**
U.S. Department of Health
and Human Services
8270 Willow Oaks Corporate Drive
Fairfax, VA 22031
Phone: 800-994-9662
TDD: 888-220-5446
Website: http://www.
womenshealth.gov/Pregnancy

Nemours Foundation
Website:
http://www.kidshealth.org
E-mail: info@kidshealth.org

Office on Women's Health
Department of Health
and Human Services
200 Independence Avenue, SW
Room 712E
Washington, DC 20201
Phone: 202-690-7650
Fax: 202-205-2631

**Planned Parenthood
Federation of America**
434 West 33rd Street
New York, NY 10001
Toll-Free: 1-800-230-PLAN (7526)
Phone: 212-541-7800
Fax: 212-245-1845
Website:
http://www.plannedparenthood.org

**Sexuality Information and
Education Council of the United
States (SIECUS)**
90 John St. Suite 402
New York, NY 10038
Phone: 212-819-9770
Fax: 212-819-9776
Website: http://www.siecus.org
E-mail: siecus@siecus.org

Social Health Education
7162 Reading Road, Suite 702
Cincinnati, OH 45237
Phone: 513-924-1444
Fax: 513-924-1434
Website: http://
www.socialhealtheducation.org

tSTD Services Group Inc.
10 South Riverside Plaza
Suite 1800
Chicago, IL 60606
Phone: 877-242-8710
Website: http://www.tstd.org
E-mail: info@tstd.org

U.S. Department of Health and Human Services (HHS)
200 Independence Avenue, SW
Washington, DC 20201
Toll-Free: 877-696-6775
Phone: 202-619-0257
Website: http://www.hhs.gov

U.S. Food and Drug Administration (FDA)
10903 New Hampshire Ave.
Silver Spring, MD 20993-0002
Toll-Free: 888-INFO-FDA
(888-463-6332)
Website: http://www.fda.gov

Chapter 72

Additional Reading About Sexuality And Sexual Health

Books

Adolescence
By Barbara Sheen
Published by Heinemann Library,
©2008
ISBN: 9781403496911

Do Abstinence Programs Work?
By Christina Fisanick
Published by Greenhaven Press,
©2010
ISBN: 9780737742923

Doing It Right
By Bronwen Pardes
Published by Simon Pulse, 2007
ISBN: 9781416918233

Endometriosis
By Stephanie Watson
Published by Rosen Pub. Group,
2007
ISBN: 9781404209046

Frequently Asked Questions About AIDS And HIV
By Richard Robinson
Published by Rosen Pub., 2009
ISBN: 9781404218086

Friendship, Dating, And Relationships
By Simone Payment
Published by Rosen Pub., 2010
ISBN: 9781435835788

About This Chapter: This chapter includes a compilation of various resources from many sources deemed reliable. It serves as a starting point for further research and is not intended to be comprehensive. Inclusion does not constitute endorsement. Resources in this chapter are categorized by type and, under each type, they are listed alphabetically by title to make topics easier to identify.

The Girl's Body Book
By Kelli S Dunham; Laura Tallardy
Published by Applesauce Press,
©2008
ISBN: 9781604330045

Hepatitis B
By Jeri Freedman
Published by Rosen Pub., 2009
ISBN: 9781435850583

Home And Family Relationships
By Tamra Orr
Published by Rosen Pub., 2010
ISBN: 9781435835795

It's Perfectly Normal: A Book About Changing Bodies, Growing Up, Sex And Sexual Health
By Robie H Harris; Michael Emberley
Published by Candlewick Press,
©2009
ISBN: 9780763644833

Ovarian Tumors And Cysts
By Tamra Orr
Published by Rosen Pub. Group,
©2009
ISBN: 9781435850606

Pelvic Inflammatory Disease (PID)
By Michael R Wilson
Published by Rosen Pub., 2009
ISBN: 9781435850590

Sexually Transmitted Diseases
By L K Currie-McGhee
Published by ReferencePoint Press,
©2009
ISBN: 9781601520456

The Truth About Abuse
By John Haley; Wendy Stein;
Heath Dingwell; Robert N Golden;
Fred L Peterson
Published by Facts On File, ©2010
ISBN: 9780816076291

The Truth About Sexual Behavior And Unplanned Pregnancy
By Elissa Howard-Barr; Fred L
Peterson; Robert N Golden; Stacey
Barrineau
Published by Facts On File, ©2009
ISBN: 9780816076345

The "What's Happening To My Body?" Book For Boys
By Lynda Madaras; Area Madaras;
Simon Sullivan
Published by: Newmarket Press,
©2007
ISBN: 9781557047694

The "What's Happening To My Body?" Book For Girls
By Area Madaras; Simon Sullivan
Published by Newmarket Press,
©2007
ISBN: 9781557047687

Articles

"Adolescent First Sex and Subsequent Mental Health," by Ann M Meier, *American Journal of Sociology*, May 2007, vol. 112, no. 6, p. 1811–1847.

"Clueless About the Risks of Oral Sex," by Bernadine Healy, *U.S. News & World Report*, 144, no. 7, 2008: 60.

"Could Hollywood Trick You Into Getting Pregnant? What TV and Movies Get Way Wrong About Sex," *Seventeen*, May 2010: 152.

"Culture: No Teen Oral-Sex 'Epidemic' After All," *Newsweek*, June 09, 2008: 55.

"Does Watching Sex on Television Predict Teen Pregnancy? Findings From a National Longitudinal Survey of Youth," by A Chandra; SC Martino; RL Collins; MN Elliott; SH Berry; DE Kanouse; A Miu, *Pediatrics*, 2008 Nov; 122(5): 1047–54.

"Exploring the Relationship Among Weight, Race, and Sexual Behaviors Among Girls," by AY Akers; CP Lynch; MA Gold; JC Chang; W Doswell; HC Wiesenfeld; W Feng; J Bost, *Pediatrics*, 2009 Nov, 124(5) e913–20.

"Health: Sex Ed—Find out Everything You Need to Know About Safe Sex," *Seventeen*, (March 2007): 110.

"How to End the War Over Sex Ed," by A Sullivan-Anderson, *Time*, 2009 Mar 30; 173(12): 40–3.

"The Myths of Teen Sex," by J Yabroff, *Newsweek*, 2008 Jun 9; 151(23): 55.

"Online Sex Offenders Prey on At-Risk Teens," by Bruce Bower, *Science News* 173, no. 8, 2008: 118.

"Patient Teenagers? A Comparison of the Sexual Behavior of Virginity Pledgers and Matched Nonpledgers," by JE Rosenbaum, *Pediatrics*, 2009 Jan; 123(1): e110–20.

"Scary Sex Rumors! Here's The Info You Need to Make Better Decisions About Your Body," *Seventeen*, September 2010: 152.

"Science: Surprising Findings on Teen Sex," *Newsweek*, November 26, 2007: 52.

"Sex and the Teenage Girl," by B D Whitehead, *Commonweal*, 135, no. 3, February 15, 2008: 8.

"Sex, Your Body, and Your Heart—Before You Hook Up, Make Sure You're Ready in Every Way," *Seventeen*, March 2009: 82.

"Society: Sex Education—Some Schools Are Finding a Middle Way Between Abstinence and Safe Sex," *Time*, March 30, 2009: 40.

"Teen Sex in America," by R Doyle, *Scientific American*, 2007 Jan; 296(1): 30.

"Throat Cancer Linked to Virus Spread by Sex," by Nathan Seppa, *Science News* 171, no. 19, 2007): 291.

"The Truth About Sex on TV—The Lies Your Favorite Shows Are Telling You, Plus How to Feel Good and Be Safe," *Seventeen* 93, January 2010: 104.

"Your Most Personal Sex Questions—There's No Question Too Embarrassing. We Won't Judge You!" *Seventeen*, February 2010: 71.

Index

Index

Page numbers that appear in *Italics* refer to tables or illustrations. Page numbers that have a small 'n' after the page number refer to information shown as Notes at the beginning of each chapter. Page numbers that appear in **Bold** refer to information contained in boxes on that page (except Notes information at the beginning of each chapter).